Managing Cancer and Living Meaningfully

An Evidence-Based Intervention for Cancer Patients and Their Caregivers

MANAGING CANCER AND LIVING MEANINGFULLY

An Evidence-Based Intervention for Cancer Patients and Their Caregivers

Gary Rodin, MD
Professor of Psychiatry and Director,
Global Institute of Psychosocial, Palliative and End-of-Life Care (GIPPEC),
Princess Margaret Cancer Centre and University of Toronto;
Joint University of Toronto/University Health Network
Harold and Shirley Lederman Chair in Psychosocial Oncology and Palliative Care;
Director of Cancer Experience, University Health Network;
Senior Scientist and Psychiatrist,
Department of Supportive Care,
Princess Margaret Cancer Centre,
University Health Network,
Toronto, Canada

Sarah Hales, MD, PhD
Psychiatrist,
Department of Supportive Care,
Princess Margaret Cancer Centre and
Centre for Mental Health, University Health Network;
Assistant Professor,
Department of Psychiatry, University of Toronto,
Toronto, Canada

OXFORD
UNIVERSITY PRESS

Oxford University Press is a department of the University of Oxford. It furthers
the University's objective of excellence in research, scholarship, and education
by publishing worldwide. Oxford is a registered trade mark of Oxford University
Press in the UK and certain other countries.

Published in the United States of America by Oxford University Press
198 Madison Avenue, New York, NY 10016, United States of America.

© Oxford University Press 2021

Library of Congress Cataloging-in-Publication Data
Title: Managing Cancer and Living Meaningfully: An Evidence-Based Intervention for Cancer
Patients and Their Caregivers By Gary Rodin, Sarah Hales.
Description: New York, NY : Oxford University Press, [2021] |
Includes bibliographical references and index.
Identifiers: LCCN 2020042690 (print) | LCCN 2020042691 (ebook) |
ISBN 9780190236427 (hardback) | ISBN 9780190236441 (epub) |
ISBN 9780190236458 (online)
Subjects: MESH: Neoplasms—psychology | Terminal Care—psychology |
Palliative Care—psychology | Advance Care Planning—standards
Classification: LCC RC271.M4 (print) | LCC RC271.M4 (ebook) |
NLM QZ 260 | DDC 616.99/40651—dc23
LC record available at https://lccn.loc.gov/2020042690
LC ebook record available at https://lccn.loc.gov/2020042691

DOI: 10.1093/med/9780190236427.001.0001

For our CALM patients and their families, whose generosity, courage and openness have taught us so much about how to live in the face of adversity

ABOUT THE COVER

As an artist, I've always been inspired by contrasts and opposing yet complementary forces. For a painter trained in the Western figurative tradition, the most dominant design imperative is the play of light against shadow masses, also known as chiaroscuro. We learn early on that the melody of light can only be expressed and fully appreciated when seen in relation to the darks. While painting at Selong Beach on the Indonesian island of Lombok, I was inspired by the dramatic effect a passing storm provided when the first rays of light began to illuminate the beach. The figures on the beach seemed to be bathed in the hopefulness that the emerging sunlight represents. This is the feeling I attempted to capture.

—John Varriano

CONTENTS

FOREWORD

CAMILLA ZIMMERMANN

Advanced cancer has become the most common cause of death in high- and middle-income countries and is one of the leading causes of death world-wide. Unlike other major causes of death, such as cardiovascular disease, end-organ failure, and neurodegenerative diseases, there is a distinct point at which cancer may be diagnosed as incurable. From an oncological perspective, this is the point at which elimination of cancer is no longer the goal, and palliative lines of anticancer treatment may begin. From a psychological perspective, this is the point when mortality is brought into sharp relief, resulting in reactions of fear, anxiety, and traumatic stress. Physical symptoms may or may not be a prominent concern, but a universal psychological task becomes preparing for the certainty of death while simultaneously engaging meaningfully in daily life. To assist and support patients in this dual psychological task, termed "double awareness," Gary Rodin and Sarah Hales developed Managing Cancer and Living Meaningfully, known by its acronym of CALM.

CALM is uniquely situated within palliative and supportive care. It was developed at the Princess Margaret Cancer Centre, in Toronto, Canada, in parallel with a more general team-based early palliative care intervention conceived by our palliative care team. At that time, I was Director of the Division of Palliative Care at the Princess Margaret Cancer Centre, while Gary was Department Head for the Department of Supportive Care. I had many conversations with Gary and Sarah about mutual patients, as well as about our respective ideas. As close collaborators in research program development and in clinical care for almost two decades, our perspectives have naturally influenced each other. Both CALM and early palliative care were developed specifically for patients with cancer, although they may be applied in a modified way to other illnesses that are life-limiting or life-threatening. Both consist of strategies to deal proactively with the challenges posed for patients and caregivers who are faced with advanced illness, and both provide whole-person care, focused on the person with the illness, rather than on the illness itself. Indeed, CALM may be considered the psychological arm of early palliative care.

Early palliative care has been a core focus of my research and clinical practice for the past two decades. Palliative care originated in the hospice movement in the 1960s and was traditionally focused on the final days and weeks of life. However, our team and others have shown that when palliative care is initiated early, from the diagnosis of advanced disease, it results in improved quality of life, symptom control, and satisfaction with medical care. Early palliative care differs from traditional palliative care in that it is delivered proactively early in the disease course, rather than reactively late in the course of illness. The initial focus is on the development of a supportive, trusting relationship with a palliative care team that provides patients and their families with emotional and practical support and assistance with decision-making. Symptoms are addressed before they become severe, and planning for the end of life is conducted when the patient and family feel comfortable doing so. Core principles of early palliative care are that it is family-centred, delivered by an interdisciplinary team, and delivered in a flexible, attentive manner focused on the needs of the patient.

When early palliative care is first initiated, the patient may have few or no physical symptoms. This lack of symptoms may be disconcerting for some palliative care practitioners, as the management of physical symptoms has traditionally been a "bridge" to an eventual discussion of psychosocial and existential concerns. CALM has filled this gap by offering a roadmap to discuss and address these important nonphysical dimensions of illness, helping patients and their caregivers face the challenges of advanced disease. Although approaches to physical symptom management are well delineated in palliative care textbooks, as is the pharmacological management of psychological distress, an organized approach to the psychotherapeutic management of psychological and existential concerns has been lacking. CALM provides a structured, although flexible approach to address these important dimensions of palliative care, centered around improving communication with healthcare providers, managing changes in self and relations with close others, reconsidering sources of meaning and purpose in life, and facing mortality while engaging meaningfully in life.

CALM can be delivered not only by psychiatrists, psychologists, and palliative care specialists but can also be taught to any professional care provider who interacts with patients with advanced cancer and their caregivers. Indeed, CALM is highly scalable. In tertiary care settings, it is useful as a psychotherapeutic intervention for psychiatrists, psychologists, social workers, and other mental health professionals providing care for those with moderate to profound distress. At the other end of the therapeutic spectrum, CALM may provide a valuable framework for providers of frontline cancer care, such as nurses, family physicians, or oncologists, to help patients cope with common reactions of grief and anxiety resulting from a diagnosis of an advanced incurable illness. CALM is a teachable, brief, evidence-based intervention that can be readily integrated into routine cancer care for anyone facing advanced disease. This scalability and relevance for multiple professions has undoubtedly contributed to the success of CALM internationally.

The wide cross-cultural applicability of CALM is evidenced by its uptake in more than 15 countries, including at centers in Europe, North and South America, Australia, and Asia. This may at first be surprising, as cultural practices surrounding death and dying vary substantially among countries and regions. However, Toronto, where CALM was conceptualized, is recognized as one of the most multicultural cities in the world, and the applicability of CALM to people of wide cultural backgrounds was an important consideration in its development. Moreover, although discussion of death and even of cancer may be taboo in some countries, individual fears and worries regarding responsiveness of cancer to treatment, physical symptoms, dependency, and mortality are universal. CALM provides a structure for conversations that may otherwise be daunting and offers guidance in navigating the course of a serious illness within a broad range of sociocultural landscapes.

It is important to mention that both Gary and Sarah are accomplished researchers in addition to being skilled therapists. Accordingly, the evidence base for CALM has been developed systematically through rigorous quantitative and qualitative research. This has culminated in the publication of a definitive phase III randomized controlled trial in the *Journal of Clinical Oncology* demonstrating the benefits of CALM compared to usual care alone.

This book is indispensable as a detailed treatment manual for those who wish to incorporate CALM into their clinical practice. However, it is also an exposition of the theoretical underpinnings of CALM, supported by years of careful research. I congratulate the authors on this remarkable work, which will undoubtedly improve the lives of patients and caregivers faced with advanced cancer across the globe for generations to come.

PREFACE

This text is the product of partnerships and relationships fostered over the past two decades. It started with our shared interest in human experience and our ambition to relieve suffering through psychotherapeutic interventions. What was initially a supervisor–supervisee relationship transformed over the years into a full partnership that led to the creation of the Managing Cancer and Living Meaningfully intervention, referred to as CALM. CALM was, in fact, the crystallization of principles and concepts that we had been developing in our work together and applying to the problem of advanced cancer. While there are many unique aspects to the problem of advanced disease, CALM is, in some respects, intended to address fundamental human dilemmas related to life's finitude and meaning.

So many have made essential contributions to the CALM clinical, research, and training program. Chris Lo, a research psychologist with expertise in measure development and psychometrics, research methodology, and data analysis and interpretation, was a key partner in developing the CALM research program and was instrumental in the conduct of the clinical trials that established the evidence base for CALM. Rinat Nissim, a psychologist and colleague in the Department of Supportive Care at the Princess Margaret Cancer Centre, led the qualitative studies of CALM, providing valuable information about the experience and benefit of CALM in the words of those who received it. The CALM program has equally been supported by Madeline Li, a psychiatrist and Lead of the Division of Psychosocial Oncology within the Princess Margaret Department of Supportive Care, who trained and supervised our research staff in how to identify depression in the context of advanced disease, and has led initiatives in implementing routine distress screening and evidence-based interventions at our centre. Our Research Program Manager, Anne Rydall, has over the last 20 years provided invaluable oversight and continuous support to our team of research coordinators and analysts, graduate students, and volunteers. CALM has benefited enormously from the valuable contributions of so many students, volunteers, and research staff of the Princess Margaret Cancer Centre, including Carmine Malfitano, Judy Jung, Aubrey Chiu, Tania Panday, Danielle Petricone-Westwood, Sarah Watt, Eryn Tong, and Ekaterina An. The first group of trained Princess Margaret CALM therapists, including social workers Valerie Heller, Cheryl Kanter, Rhonda Kibrick-Lazear, Fiorella Lubertacci, and Jenny Shaheed, psychiatrist Peter Fitzgerald, and advanced practice nurses Kelly McGuigan, Maurene McQuestion, and Patricia Murphy-Kane, were involved in early CALM trials and openly shared their experiences in CALM therapy to inform and shape CALM and our training model. CALM has also benefited from the many students, volunteers, and staff of the Princess Margaret Department of Supportive Care and the Global Institute of Psychosocial, Palliative, and End-of-Life Care (GIPPEC) who have devoted their time and effort over the years to administrative and research activities that have helped make CALM what it is today. In addition to our CALM research staff named above, we are most grateful to Lesley Chalklin, GIPPEC Program Manager, Joanna Shnall, Alanna Chu, and Twinkle Arora, who have been essential to the global dissemination of CALM and to maintaining our linkages with our international colleagues. Finally, the enthusiastic engagement of a large international community in the Global CALM program has been, for us, an unexpected pleasure. Our international collaborations, which are described in more depth in Chapter 12 and in the epilogue, have been personally meaningful and have supported the Global CALM program by deepening our understanding of CALM's applicability across cultures.

CALM was born in part from our partnership with Camilla Zimmermann, with whom we worked to help build the Department of Supportive Care at the Princess Margaret Cancer Centre. We shared a vision—now realized—for a department that would include psychosocial oncology, palliative care, and cancer rehabilitation and survivorship and in which research would be fully integrated with clinical care and education. Camilla has been a pioneer in the integration of palliative care in oncology and in conducting rigorous research to demonstrate its effectiveness. We developed CALM within this context, adding structure, training, and evidence to the psychological dimensions of early palliative care. It has also benefited greatly from the support of the Princess Margaret Cancer Centre, the Princess Margaret Cancer Foundation, the Conjoint University of Toronto/University Health Network Harold and Shirley Lederman Chair in Psychosocial Oncology and Palliative Care, the University Health Network Centre for Mental Health, the Canadian Institutes of Health Research, and Movember, the international cancer-focused charity that is based in Melbourne, Australia. We are most grateful for the support that we have received at all stages of the process in the development of the CALM program.

We hope, through this text, to enrich your understanding of the impact of cancer and to provide insight into the opportunities to relieve distress and promote psychological well-being through a psychotherapeutic intervention such as CALM. Although much has been accomplished in the CALM program, the years to come will see continued efforts to further our understanding of the therapeutic process, refine our measurement tools, gather additional evidence in international settings, understand any cultural modifications that may be required, train therapists and CALM supervisors throughout the world, and improve access to CALM through online and other platforms. We look forward to hearing from you about your observations, reflections, and experiences with the problem of advanced cancer and the CALM intervention.

ACKNOWLEDGMENTS

The authors wish to acknowledge the invaluable editorial assistance of members of our research team, especially Anne Barbeau, as well as Anne Rydall, Eryn Tong, and Twinkle Arora, and the support of Andrea Knobloch and Jacqueline Buckley of Oxford University Press at all stages in the process of publication.

CONTRIBUTORS

Ekaterina An, MSc
Clinical Research Coordinator,
  Department of Supportive Care,
  Princess Margaret Cancer Centre,
  University Health Network, and
  Global Institute of Psychosocial,
  Palliative and End-of-Life Care,
  Princess Margaret Cancer Centre
  and University of Toronto,
  Toronto, Canada
(Chapters 8 & 9)

Jennifer Bell, PhD
Bioethicist, Department of
  Supportive Care, Princess Margaret
  Cancer Centre, University Health
  Network;
Assistant Professor, Department of
  Psychiatry, and Member, Joint
  Centre for Bioethics, University of
  Toronto, Toronto, Canada
(Chapter 6)

Alanna Chu, MPH
Clinical Research Analyst,
  Department of Supportive Care,
  Princess Margaret Cancer Centre,
  University Health Network, and
  Global Institute of Psychosocial,
  Palliative and End-of-Life Care,
  Princess Margaret Cancer Centre
  and University of Toronto,
  Toronto, Canada
(Chapter 12)

Froukje de Vries, MD, PhD
Psychiatrist, Department of
  Supportive Care, Princess Margaret
  Cancer Centre, University Health
  Network, Toronto, Canada;
  Department of Psychiatry
  and Centre for Quality of Life,
  Netherlands Cancer Institute,
  Amsterdam, The Netherlands
(Chapter 10)

Carmine Malfitano, MSW, RSW
Social Worker in Research,
Department of Supportive Care,
  Princess Margaret Cancer Centre,
  University Health Network;
Research Associate, Global Institute
  of Psychosocial, Palliative and End-
  of-Life Care, Princess Margaret
  Cancer Centre and University of
  Toronto, Toronto, Canada;
PhD candidate, University of Ferrara,
  Ferrara, Italy
(Chapters 2 & 9)

Rinat Nissim, PhD, CPsych
Clinical Psychologist, Department of
  Supportive Care, Princess Margaret
  Cancer Centre, University Health
  Network;
Assistant Professor, Department of
  Psychiatry, University of Toronto,
  Toronto, Canada
(Chapter 3)

Gilla K. Shapiro, MA (Cantab),
  MPP/MPA, PhD, CPsych
Postdoctoral Fellow,
Department of Supportive Care,
Princess Margaret Cancer Centre,
  University Health Network,
  Toronto, Canada
(Chapter 7)

Chloe Shaw, PhD, MRes
Honorary Research Associate,
Neonatology, Institute for Women's
  Health, London, England
(Chapter 5)

Introduction

The Walking Wounded

Waiting to die is no way to live.

—CALM participant

Advances in medical treatment and changing demographics mean that a growing number of individuals in the world are living with advanced cancer. They are the *walking wounded*, facing the threat of impending mortality and the challenge of continuing with their lives. Their task differs from those who are at the end of life, whose primary goal is to face death with comfort and equanimity. The latter is no small accomplishment, but living meaningfully in the face of advanced disease is, in some respects, an even greater challenge.

Developing a text on psychotherapy for individuals with cancer facing the threat of impending mortality is a daunting task. Such an undertaking touches on the worlds of oncology, palliative care, psychology, psychotherapy, and existential philosophy, each of which has their own vast literature and universe of discourse, with relatively little interdisciplinary sharing of knowledge, experience, or practical applications. The ambitious and perhaps unachievable intent of this book is to bridge these fields and provide a roadmap for therapists and patients to address the challenges of advanced disease.

The book begins with the psychological and social dimensions of advanced cancer, drawing upon decades of clinical experience and research conducted by our team and by others. We have conducted qualitative and quantitative studies of more than 1,000 individuals and their families living with *advanced* or *metastatic* cancer (see Chapter 3 of this volume). These designations refer broadly to cancer that is progressive and threatens to shorten life, but with which meaningful life may still be possible. Although none of us knows which will be the last year of our life, the diagnosis of advanced cancer brings this uncertainty into uncomfortable awareness. Disease of this kind is an "unwelcome intruder" into the lives of those affected, as was described almost a century ago by Sigmund Freud, who suffered from an oropharyngeal cancer for more than 15 years before it took his life (Romm, 1983). Despite the presence of this cancer, the years after Freud was diagnosed were some of his most meaningful and productive. Managing Cancer and Living Meaningfully (CALM) is an evidence-based intervention developed by our team to help patients and their caregivers effectively manage the challenges, tasks, and crises triggered by advanced disease and to live their lives as meaningfully as possible.

OUR PATH TO CALM

We began our work in cancer at the Princess Margaret Cancer Centre in Toronto, Canada, more than two decades ago, searching for ways to better support patients with advanced cancer and their caregivers. We found that patients were immersed and sometimes lost in the world of cancer treatment, struggling to maintain "dual citizenship, in the kingdom of the well and the kingdom of the sick" (Sontag, 1978, p. 3). We aimed to identify factors in these individuals, in their family environment, and in the cancer treatment setting that would either support them in their new circumstances or put them at risk. We examined the influence of such factors as attachment security and spiritual well-being and reformulated traditional concepts of death anxiety, death awareness, death acceptance, and the will to live. Drawing upon our empirical observations and the theoretical frameworks of attachment, relational, and terror management theories, we reconceptualized the psychology of impending mortality and developed a clinical intervention aimed at reducing distress and fostering growth in those facing advanced disease.

WHAT IS CALM?

CALM is a semi-structured, supportive-expressive psychotherapeutic intervention that can be as brief as three to six sessions. It is designed to provide a framework and reflective space for patients to consider the practical and profound issues that arise with advanced cancer. Although advanced cancer may affect patients and their families in a myriad of ways, there are common and prototypical challenges which this condition presents for them. CALM helps clinicians address four distinct but interrelated domains that reflect the challenges and opportunities that individuals with advanced cancer most often face. These are:

1. *Symptom management and communication with healthcare providers*, which involves exploration of patients' physical symptoms and functioning, their relationships with their healthcare providers, and their participation in their care and in medical decision-making. Relationships with healthcare providers are critically important for patients facing advanced disease due to symptoms that require careful and balanced management, the life-and-death treatment decisions that must be made, and ongoing disease-related concerns. Patients are increasingly encouraged to share in decision-making, but due to the complexity of treatment decisions and the ambiguity of the evidence, trusting relationships with healthcare providers are essential for this to occur. Developing these relationships of trust with healthcare providers is an enormous challenge for many patients, particularly because clinic visits are often brief and focused much more on the disease and its symptoms than on the patient's values and experience. The CALM therapist creates a safe space for patients to clarify the values and beliefs that may influence their treatment decisions (see Chapter 6 of this volume) and to discuss relationships and communication with their healthcare team.

2. *Changes in self and relations with close others*, which includes helping patients maintain or reclaim their sense of self and core identity. Advanced disease may undermine their body image, functional capacity, and ability to engage in meaningful activities. The heightened dependency brought on by the disease also constitutes an enormous threat to many individuals with advanced cancer. Those who have tended to be self-reliant, autonomous, and more comfortable in a caregiving role now must accept vulnerability and dependency on others. Those who worry about the availability of support may become highly distressed. The CALM therapist must attend to attachment security (see Chapter 4 of this volume) and help patients renegotiate important attachment relationships in the context of advanced disease.

3. *Spirituality and the sense of meaning and purpose in life*, which refers to the patient's values, beliefs, sense of meaning, goals, and priorities in

the context of a shortened lifespan. The perceived shortness of time heightens the need to reconsider what is or can be meaningful in life, and the reflective space provided in CALM can support these shifts in meaning and priorities. CALM is intended to help patients make sense of their lives and their current situations and to understand how their past experiences have shaped the present experience of their disease. It may lead to a positive sense of legacy, but this may first require acceptance and validation of regrets and disappointments about their lives. Empathic understanding of these difficult feelings by the therapist may allow some individuals to reclaim and integrate more positive dimensions of their past and present lives.

4. *Preparing for the future, sustaining hope, and facing mortality*, which includes exploring attitudes and fears about dying and death, as well as planning for the future and the end of life. CALM sessions can provide a safe place in which these sensitive and important conversations can begin, particularly for patients who fear that such discussions will inordinately burden or distress their families. Concerns that emerge in relation to the end of life may relate to the sense that important life goals have not been achieved, that there is a lack of closure in their important relationships, that their close others will be burdened by their demise, or that their death will be sudden or painful. Uncertainty about the future may not only generate enormous distress but may also create a "now moment" (Stern et al., 1998) in which patients can rethink the life that they have lived and that which they can live in the time that remains.

The four CALM domains are reminders or signposts for therapists of the issues that are commonly important to patients with advanced disease and for which opportunities should be created for discussion. These domains help to structure the purpose of CALM, an important aspect of brief psychotherapy (Malan, 1976), although the sequence and priority of each domain will vary with each patient and session. We initially referred to these domains as "modules," but found that this term implied to some a fixed sequence in which they should be addressed. For that reason, we relabeled them as "domains," a term that seemed to better represent the broad and often interrelated areas of focus. This is more consistent with the aim of the CALM therapist to follow the narrative of the patient, rather than to adhere to a fixed sequence of topics. The need for variability in the sequence of CALM domains became particularly evident when we examined the emergence of issues related to mortality, the fourth domain.

We had expected, given the sensitive nature of mortality-related fears, that issues in this domain would not appear until near the end of therapy or later in the course of the disease. However, we found that mortality-related concerns commonly emerged early in the first session in response to open-ended questioning by the therapist, even without specific prompting (Shaw et al., 2017).

The therapeutic relationship in CALM is the foundation upon which the entire endeavor depends. Therapists aim to provide a secure base and to be curious and open to the experience of patients, supporting their courage to explore new ways and new modes of being in the world. The CALM therapist offers interpretations tentatively, with the intent to create new meanings jointly with the patient. CALM aims to support "double awareness," a concept elaborated by our team in which life engagement is sustained alongside planning for the limitations of the disease and the end of life (Rodin & Zimmermann, 2008; see Chapter 5 of this volume). Sustaining this duality in the context of advanced disease is a very different goal than that implied by the more linear progression from protest and denial to acceptance outlined in some earlier models of adjustment to the end of life (Kübler-Ross, 1969; see Chapter 3 of this volume). CALM also fits squarely within the modern view of the therapeutic process as the joint construction of a mutually meaningful narrative (Atwood & Stolorow, 1984), rather than the discovery of historical truth (Spence, 1982). The sense of meaning and coherence derived from the creation of such personal narratives, referred to as autobiographical reasoning, is an important means by which individuals learn to manage difficult life experiences (Weststrate & Glück, 2017). The emotional presence of the CALM therapist, with attention to the modulation of affect, allows this process to be sustained, with therapists aiming to facilitate emotional expression and to diminish the numbing of emotions or the persistence of overwhelming emotional distress.

THE EVIDENCE BASE

Research conducted by our team over the past 20 years has confirmed that the will to live is almost universal in individuals who are living with advanced disease, even when they understand their prognosis and what lies ahead (e.g., Rodin et al., 2007). Notwithstanding the public interest in assisted dying in some parts of the world, this will to live seems to be "hardwired" in humans, even when the end is near. At the same time, individuals with advanced disease value empathic and honest communication with their medical caregivers about their disease and their prognosis (Rodin,

Mackay, et al., 2009). Such communication is essential for them to make informed decisions in the complex and challenging context of advanced disease. Well-intentioned efforts of families and healthcare providers to protect cancer patients from being aware of the seriousness of their condition may only increase their sense of isolation. Psychological adjustment in this situation depends not on avoiding the unavoidable, but on processing feelings of loss and grief that may be profound, finding new sources of meaning, accepting the requirements of growing dependency, and preserving the sense of self, despite the ravages of disease. CALM was designed to address these issues.

The evidence base that led to the development of CALM and the scientific framework in which we evaluated its effectiveness have contributed greatly to its acceptance within the oncology and supportive care communities. Beginning with the longitudinal Will to Live study in 2007, we demonstrated that symptoms of depression and demoralization are common in individuals with advanced cancer and often worsen with greater proximity to the end of life (Lo et al., 2010; see Chapter 3 of this volume). We applied and tested terror management theory (see Chapter 2 of this volume) to better understand the factors that might protect against or put patients at risk for this distress. Consistent with this theory, we demonstrated that three psychological pillars—self-esteem, attachment security, and the sense of meaning in life—protected individuals with advanced disease from depression and demoralization (Rodin, Lo, et al., 2009). CALM was designed to strengthen these pillars and help patients with advanced disease to manage the hurdles that they will inevitably face.

Our randomized controlled trial of CALM gave further scientific credibility to the clinical observations that had been emerging about its impact. The trial demonstrated that CALM is effective in relieving and preventing symptoms of depression at both three and six months (see Chapters 7 and 10 of this volume; Rodin et al., 2018). It also showed that CALM relieves and prevents distress about death and dying in those who have moderate levels of such distress at baseline. Individuals who received CALM reported feeling better prepared for the end of life. Finally, those receiving CALM reported significantly greater benefit on all CALM-specific dimensions of well-being than did those receiving usual care alone (see Chapter 10 of this volume).

The psychological states of patients with advanced disease cannot be disentangled from the world of cancer in which they live. This assumption is fundamental to CALM, which is intended to be fully integrated with cancer care and palliative care. Therapists who are embedded in and understand the world of cancer have unique value in this circumstance. Their circumscribed role affords them the time and space to address in depth the psychological issues that typically cannot be addressed in either palliative care or cancer care, where multiple other tasks must be performed by the practitioners of these disciplines.

STRUCTURE OF THE BOOK

This text is written for healthcare providers of all disciplines who wish to understand more about the psychology of advanced disease and how to intervene more effectively to help those living with life-threatening illness. It may also be of value to patients and caregivers who are interested in a deeper understanding of these issues.

Part I of the book begins with an exploration of the theoretical frameworks and research that informed the development of CALM. CALM emerged in the context of transformative developments in medicine and in our understanding of the mind. The works of Heinz Kohut (1977), John Bowlby (1969), Stephen Mitchell (2000), Elisabeth Kübler-Ross (1969), Barney Glaser and Anselm Strauss (1965), E. Mansell Pattison (1977), and Dame Cicely Saunders (2001) were foundational to the development of CALM. These pioneers helped to shift views in psychotherapy, medicine, and end-of-life care from more positivist models to ones more squarely focused on human subjectivity and its empathic understanding. CALM also arose, as did other dimensions of early palliative care, in response to the more prolonged survival of patients with advanced disease enabled by newer treatment modalities.

Part II of this book contains the CALM manual, which presents the specific content and process of the CALM intervention for those who wish to learn more about its delivery. It outlines the practical application of CALM both for those new to the intervention and those more experienced with CALM therapy.

We hope that the text will provide both new and familiar ways of understanding how to help individuals with advanced disease to live as well as possible in the time that remains. We have sought in this work to open a window into the inner and outer worlds of those living with a life-threatening illness, which we believe has far-reaching implications for the human condition and for how each of us choose to live our lives. We are grateful that you have joined us for this journey into the lives of patients and their families facing advanced disease. We hope that we can convey at least some of the power, poignancy, and privilege of being able to work with individuals at this most difficult moment in their lives. We hope that this text will encourage you to engage in this work and in the global project we have undertaken to help patients with advanced disease and their families manage cancer and live meaningfully.

REFERENCES

Atwood, G., & Stolorow, R. (1984). *Structures of subjectivity: Explorations in psychoanalytic phenomenology.* The Analytic Press.

Bowlby, J. (1969). *Attachment and loss.* Vol. I: *Attachment.* Hogarth Press and the Institute of Psycho-Analysis.

Glaser, B. G., & Strauss, A. L. (1965). *Awareness of dying.* Aldine Transaction.

Kohut, H. (1977). *The restoration of the self.* International Universities Press, Inc.

Kübler-Ross, E. (1969). *On death and dying.* Tavistock Publications.

Lo, C., Zimmermann, C., Rydall, A., Walsh, A., Jones, J. M., Moore, M. J., Shepherd, F. A., Gagliese, L., & Rodin, G. (2010). Longitudinal study of depressive symptoms in patients with metastatic gastrointestinal and lung cancer. *Journal of Clinical Oncology, 28*(18), 3084–3089.

Malan, D. H. (1976). *The frontier of brief psychotherapy: An example of the convergence of research and clinical practice.* Plenum Medical Book Co.

Mitchell, S. A. (2000). *Relationality: From attachment to intersubjectivity.* The Analytics Press.

Pattison, E. M. (1977). *The experience of dying.* Prentice Hall.

Rodin, G., Lo, C., Mikulincer, M., Donner, A., Gagliese, L., & Zimmermann, C. (2009). Pathways to distress: The multiple determinants of depression, hopelessness, and the desire for hastened death in metastatic cancer patients. *Social Science & Medicine, 68*(3), 562–569.

Rodin, G., Lo, C., Rydall, A., Shnall, J., Malfitano, C., Chiu, A., Panday, T., Watt, S., An, E., Nissim, R., Li, M. Zimmermann, C., & Hales, S. (2018). Managing Cancer and Living Meaningfully (CALM): A randomized controlled trial of a psychological intervention for patients with advanced cancer. *Journal of Clinical Oncology, 36*(23), 2422–2432.

Rodin, G., Mackay, J. A., Zimmermann, C., Mayer, C., Howell, D., Katz, M., Sussman, J., & Brouwers, M. (2009). Clinician-patient communication: A systematic review. *Supportive Care in Cancer, 17*(6), 627–644.

Rodin, G., & Zimmermann, C. (2008). Psychoanalytic reflections on mortality: A reconsideration. *Journal of the American Academy of Psychoanalysis and Dynamic Psychiatry, 36*(1), 181–196.

Rodin, G., Zimmermann, C., Rydall, A., Jones, J., Shepherd, F. A., Moore, M., Fruh, M., Donner, A., & Gagliese, L. (2007). The desire for hastened death in patients with metastatic cancer. *Journal of Pain and Symptom Management, 33*(6), 661–675.

Romm, S. (1983). *The unwelcome intruder: Freud's struggle with cancer.* Praeger.

Saunders, C. (2001). The evolution of palliative care. *Journal of the Royal Society of Medicine, 94* (9), 430–432.

Shaw, C., Chrysikou, V., Davis, S., Gessler, S., Rodin, G., & Lanceley, A. (2017). Inviting end-of-life talk in initial CALM therapy sessions: A conversation analytic study. *Patient Education and Counseling, 100*(2), 259–266.

Sontag, S. (1978). *Illness as metaphor*. Farrar, Straus and Giroux.

Spence, D. P. (1982). *Narrative truth and historical truth: Meaning and interpretation in psychoanalysis*. W. W. Norton and Company.

Stern, D. N., Sander, L. W., Nahum, J. P., Harrison, A. M., Lyons-Ruth, K., Morgan, A. C., Bruschweiler-Stern, N., & Tronick, E. Z. (1998). Non-interpretive mechanisms in psychoanalytic therapy: The 'something more' than interpretation. *International Journal of Psycho-Analysis, 79* (Pt 5), 903–921.

Weststrate, N. M., & Glück, J. (2017). Hard-earned wisdom: Exploratory processing of difficult life experience is positively associated with wisdom. *Developmental Psychology, 53*(4), 800–814.

PART 1

CALM Foundations

CHAPTER 1

The Meaning of Mortality in Modern Life

INTRODUCTION

The last century has seen unprecedented advances in medical and public health interventions, with a doubling of global life expectancy (Roser et al., 2019). However, this has not been accompanied by a parallel investment in supporting the human dimensions of medical care for many individuals at the most difficult time of their lives. The palliative care movement and, more specifically, the Managing Cancer and Living Meaningfully (CALM) intervention emerged in response to the growing needs of this population and to the lack of sufficient attention to their suffering in modern medical care.

The relatively low priority in medicine given to the social and psychological aspects of disease has many causes, including the nature of modern medical education, the biases and priorities of decision makers in healthcare, and societal attitudes toward illness and mortality. In high-income countries, the enormous investments in biotechnology and aggressive medical interventions have not been accompanied by necessary and complementary investments in palliative and supportive care (Jordan et al., 2018). Even in low- and middle-income countries, there has often been investment in expensive medical interventions of minimal benefit without ensuring that the basic elements of medical or supportive care are in place (Sullivan et al., 2017). The prioritization of technology and aggressive interventions has often been considered as objective and self-evident, rather than reflecting "cultural systems of value in health" (Napier et al., 2014, p. 1607), in which emotional distress may be given a lower priority than other forms of suffering.

Recent decades have seen a growing voice from the public and from patients who want and expect better support in managing the burden of disease and the threat of mortality. This expectation is partly due to the secularization of many societies and the consequent loss of cultural sources of meaning. This societal shift has led many patients and their families to seek emotional support and meaning from their healthcare providers (Timmermans, 2005). Palliative care emerged in response to these needs, but even in this most humanistic field, there has been much more attention to the physical burden of disease than to its psychological and social dimensions.

The lack of training and support for healthcare providers in most parts of the world to provide effective psychological care to their patients is consistent with the tendency in modern medicine to privilege approaches that involve biology and technology over those that involve empathy (Napier et al., 2014). Empathy, almost certainly the least expensive medical intervention, is not only an innate human capacity, but also one that can be enhanced through education and modeling (Buckman et al., 2011). Empathy is a core therapeutic element of CALM.

WHY CANCER?

The so-called Emperor of All Maladies (Mukherjee, 2010), cancer has evoked fear in humans from the time of antiquity. It was once a hidden and mysterious condition but in the last century has become a central societal and medical preoccupation. Cancer is expected to become the leading cause of death in the 21st century and is the single most important barrier to greater life expectancy in every country of the world (Bray et al., 2018). The rise in the incidence and prevalence of cancer is related to multiple factors, including the aging and growth of the population, the decline in mortality related to cardiac and infectious diseases, and lifestyle changes that increase the risk of cancer (Bray et al., 2018). Further, immunotherapy and newer targeted therapies have produced prolonged remissions or have halted disease progression for many patients with less toxicity than that associated with traditional chemotherapy, resulting in more individuals living with advanced cancer. Indeed, the improved survival in these individuals is one of the most remarkable achievements in medicine in recent decades. In some cancer types, however, the reduction in mortality rates with cancer treatment has been disappointingly small and the time that remains for such individuals becomes even more precious. Patients in this situation must find ways to live meaningfully, despite the burden of disease and the possibility of its recurrence or progression.

THE LOSS OF PERSONHOOD IN CANCER CARE

Modern healthcare has become more specialized and technologized, with the frequent unintended effect of many patients feeling dehumanized in treatment settings (Høybye & Tjørnhøj-Thomsen, 2014). Appointments in cancer clinics are often brief and focused on the disease and its treatment, with little time for attention to the whole person (Sullivan et al., 2017). Some have linked this to the decline of traditional medicine, in which physicians knew their patients and their families across the life cycle and the therapeutic relationship was at the heart of clinical encounters. The specialization and technologization of medicine and the growth of the population in large urban centers has often undermined the possibility of these more personal medical relationships. Somehow, expertise in communication and rapport came to be regarded as "soft skills," not essential to study or teach, with the disturbing consequence that empathy now actually declines in modern medical trainees over the course of medical school and in subsequent residency training (Quince et al., 2016). This decline presumably results from what trainees are taught, from what they observe is practiced by those whom they respect, and from the lack of support for them to process their own experience in emotion-laden medical encounters (Buckman et al., 2011). While artificial intelligence and machine learning may lead to many advances in the diagnosis and treatment of medical conditions (Lynch & Liston, 2018; Topol, 2019), these developments are unlikely, at least in the short term, to replace the therapeutic value of human relationships in healthcare.

Clinicians also are affected by these shifts in society and in healthcare, and they often struggle to work in healthcare systems that are increasingly technologized and focused on disease-related interventions, even near the end of life. It has been suggested that the global focus on cost-effective performance has led to the progressive dehumanization of healthcare and that a shift to patient-centered health systems is needed (The Lancet [Editorial], 2019). Healthcare providers are losing the ability to connect with patients, and moral distress and burnout have been shown to be common among oncologists and other clinicians (Yates & Samuel, 2019).

THE RISE OF CONSUMER-DRIVEN HEALTHCARE

Individuals in many parts of the world are now insisting upon their participation in medical decision-making and in having their medical care directed to improve both the quality and length of their life. Patients are increasingly turning to healthcare providers for psychological support throughout the course of their disease, sometimes with great disappointment. The gap between what patients with advanced cancer want from their physicians and what they receive was highlighted by a study at a large American cancer center. This research showed that a substantial proportion of patients with advanced cancer want spiritual care to be provided by their physicians, but only a very small proportion of physicians report being adequately trained to do so (Balboni et al., 2013). To bridge this gap, much more attention is needed to the development of these skills in undergraduate, postgraduate, and continuing medical education programs (Bylund, 2017; Patel et al., 2019).

There has been increasing societal interest in issues of dying and death, which, in turn, has led to a growing demand that the healthcare system better support those with advanced disease from the time of diagnosis to the end of life. In some regions, healthy people are meeting as part of "death cafes" to discuss and confront mortality in the hopes of preparing for the inevitability of death (Miles & Corr, 2017). Popular nonfiction books such as Atul Gawande's *Being Mortal* (2014) and Paul Kalanithi's *When Breath Becomes Air* (2016) have become international bestsellers. These shifts may be related to medical advances and the more prolonged survival of those with advanced diseases and perhaps occur in reaction to the frequently dehumanizing experience of medical care.

PSYCHOLOGICAL INTERVENTIONS FOR ADVANCED CANCER

In response to these societal changes, there has been growing understanding that the care of those with advanced disease should extend to the psychological, social, and spiritual dimensions of the condition. This requires clinicians to be better trained to help patients address the enormous adjustments that are required of them (Galushko et al., 2012; Hales et al., 2014). Evidence-based psychotherapeutic approaches are emerging for patients with advanced cancer (Rodin et al., 2020; see Chapter 9 of this volume). One of these is CALM, which is uniquely integrated with cancer care and palliative care and focused as much on living in the face of advanced disease as it is on disease progression and the end of life.

THE EVOLUTION OF CALM

As mental health clinicians working in a comprehensive cancer center for more than two decades, we have been immersed in the medical world of cancer care and in the personal worlds of people living with incurable disease. We have been touched and impressed by the courage and bravery of these individuals and their families and have been struck by the commonality of the challenges that they face. Our colleagues in cancer centers throughout the world have made similar observations and have also struggled with the lack of a systematic or uniform approach to help patients and families manage the challenges of progressive cancer and live as meaningfully as possible.

We aimed to develop an intervention that could be implemented as part of standard care for patients with advanced and progressive disease. We had become convinced that the traditional approach in cancer care of waiting until patients become depressed, demoralized, or suicidal before referring them for psychological care was failing those living with this disease. Drawing on research, theory, and, most importantly, on our experience with the patients whom we saw daily in our clinics, we developed CALM. Over the last decade, the interest and enthusiasm of colleagues from all parts of the world in this approach has been overwhelming. With their help, we have now trained thousands of clinicians across the globe in CALM, many of whom return year after year to Toronto, Canada, to attend our training workshops (see Chapter 12 of this volume). Our colleagues have continued to ask for a published work that brings it all together, which led to the writing of this book.

We know that it is impossible to capture in words the poignancy and power of these human interactions, but we hope that the descriptions and case examples included in this text will convey at least some of the intimate and personal dimensions of CALM. We leave readers to judge for themselves whether such an approach could or should be an essential and standard aspect of care for patients with advanced cancer around the world. We believe that this would better serve patients and their families and perhaps engage more clinicians in the deeply satisfying task of helping patients with advanced cancer to manage their disease and to live their lives more meaningfully.

REFERENCES

Balboni, T. A., Balboni, M., Enzinger, A. C., Gallivan, K., Paulk, M. E., Wright, A., Steinhauser, K., VanderWeele, T. J., & Prigerson, H. G. (2013). Provision of spiritual support to patients with advanced cancer by religious communities and associations with medical care at the end of life. *JAMA Internal Medicine,* *173*(12), 1109–1117.
Bray, F., Ferlay, J., Soerjomataram, I., Siegel, R. L., Torre, L. A., & Jemal, A. (2018). Global cancer statistics 2018: GLOBOCAN estimates of incidence and

mortality worldwide for 36 cancers in 185 countries. *CA: A Cancer Journal for Clinicians, 68*(6), 394–424.

Buckman, R., Tulsky, J. A., & Rodin, G. (2011). Empathic responses in clinical practice: Intuition or tuition? *CMAJ: Canadian Medical Association Journal, 183*(5), 569–571.

Bylund, C. L. (2017). Taking the 'training' out of communication skills training. *Patient Education and Counseling, 100*(7), 1408–1409.

Galushko, M., Romotzky, V., & Voltz, R. (2012). Challenges in end-of-life communication. *Current Opinion in Supportive and Palliative Care, 6*(3), 355–364.

Gawande, A. (2014). *Being mortal: Ilness, medicine, and what matters in the end.* Metropolitan Books.

Hales, S., Chiu, A., Husain, A., Braun, M., Rydall, A., Gagliese, L., Zimmermann, C., & Rodin, G. (2014). The quality of dying and death in cancer and its relationship to palliative care and place of death. *Journal of Pain and Symptom Management, 48*(5), 839–851.

Høybye, M. T., & Tjørnhøj-Thomsen, T. (2014). Encounters in cancer treatment: Intersubjective configurations of a need for rehabilitation. *Medical Anthropology Quarterly, 28*(3), 305–322.

Jordan, K., Aapro, M., Kaasa, S., Ripamonti, C. I., Scotté, F., Strasser, F., Young, A., Bruera, E., Herrstedt, J., Keefe, D., Laird, B., Walsh, D., Douillard, J. Y., & Cervantes, A. (2018). European Society for Medical Oncology (ESMO) position paper on supportive and palliative care. *Annals of Oncology, 29*(1), 36–43.

Kalanithi, P. (2016). *When breath becomes air.* Random House.

Lynch, C. J., & Liston, C. (2018). New machine-learning technologies for computer-aided diagnosis. *Nature Medicine, 24*(9), 1304–1305.

Miles, L., & Corr, C. A. (2017). Death cafe: What is it and what we can learn from it. *OMEGA-Journal of Death and Dying, 75*(2), 151–165.

Mukherjee, S. (2010). *The emperor of all maladies: A biography of cancer.* Simon & Schuster.

Napier, A. D., Ancarno, C., Butler, B., Calabrese, J., Chater, A., Chatterjee, H., Guesnet, F., Horne, R., Jacyna, S., Jadhav, S., Macdonald, A., Neuendorf, U., Parkhurst, A., Reynolds, R., Scambler, G., Shamdasani, S., Smith, S. Z., Stougaard-Nielsen, J., Thomson, L., Tyler, N., Volkmann, A. M., Walker, T., Watson, J., Williams, A. C., Willott, C., Wilson, J., & Woolf, K. (2014). Culture and health. *The Lancet, 384*(9954), 1607–1639.

Patel, S., Pelletier-Bui, A., Smith, S., Roberts, M. B., Kilgannon, H., Trzeciak, S., & Roberts, B. W. (2019). Curricula for empathy and compassion training in medical education: A systematic review. *PLoS One, 14*(8), e0221412. doi: 10.1371/journal.pone.0221412.

Quince, T., Thiemann, P., Benson, J., & Hyde, S. (2016). Undergraduate medical students' empathy: Current perspectives. *Advances in Medical Education and Practice, 7*, 443–455.

Rodin, G., An, E., Shnall, J., & Malfitano, C. (2020). Psychological interventions for patients with advanced disease: Implications for oncology and palliative care. *Journal of Clinical Oncology, 38*(9), 885–904.

Roser, M., Ortiz-Ospina, E., & Ritchie, H. (2019). Life Expectancy. *Published online at OurWorldInData.org.* Retrieved from: 'https://ourworldindata.org/

life-expectancy' [Online Resource. First published in 2013; last revised in October 2019].

Sullivan, R., Pramesh, C. S., & Booth, C. M. (2017). Cancer patients need better care, not just more technology. *Nature, 549*(7672), 325–328.

The Lancet [Editorial]. (2019). Physician burnout: The need to rehumanise health systems. *Lancet, 394*(10209), 1591.

Timmermans, S. (2005). Death brokering: Constructing culturally appropriate deaths. *Sociology of Health & Illness, 27*(7), 993–1013.

Topol, E. (2019). *Deep medicine: How artificial intelligence can make healthcare human again*. Basic Books.

Yates, M., & Samuel, V. (2019). Burnout in oncologists and associated factors: A systematic literature review and meta-analysis. *European Journal of Cancer Care, 28*(3), e13094. doi: 10.1111/ecc.13094.

CHAPTER 2

The Management of Terror

The news at the beginning, with each piece of information we received—it got worse.
—CALM participant

INTRODUCTION

A fundamental goal of Managing Cancer and Living Meaningfully (CALM) is to help patients and families manage the terror evoked by the diagnosis and subsequent course of metastatic cancer. States of depression and demoralization are common as the disease progresses, but anxiety and fear are most often the immediate psychological response to the shock of bad news. This response can be profound and all-encompassing, with the severity of the symptoms meeting diagnostic criteria for acute stress disorder (ASD) and, when persistent, for posttraumatic stress disorder (PTSD). In this chapter, we will describe the traumatic states that may emerge following the diagnosis, progression, or recurrence of advanced cancer and the unique contribution of CALM therapy to their relief.

TRAUMA- AND STRESSOR-RELATED DISORDERS

The exposure to a traumatic event may cause marked psychological distress, which is categorized in the *Diagnostic and Statistical Manual of Mental Disorders–Fifth Edition* (DSM-5; American Psychiatric Association [APA], 2013) under trauma- and stressor-related disorders. These states are common following physical and sexual assaults and accidents (Shalev et al.,

2017). ASD and PTSD following trauma typically present with a number of symptoms, which include:

1. *Intrusive psychological symptoms*, which may arise in dreams, memories, or dissociative flashbacks of the trauma and may manifest as intense and prolonged psychological distress or physiological reactions when exposed to reminders of the traumatic event;
2. The *avoidance of stimuli related to the traumatic event*, which involves deliberate attempts to avoid internal and external reminders of the trauma;
3. *Altered mood or cognition*, which may include self-blame, persistent negative emotions or an inability to experience positive emotions, decreased interest in significant activities, feelings of detachment from others, an inability to remember details of the traumatic event, and exaggerated negative beliefs about the self, others, or the world; and
4. *Marked arousal and reactivity*, which may manifest as irritability or anger, recklessness or self-destructive behaviors, hypervigilance, decreased concentration, an exaggerated startle response, and problems with sleep (APA, 2013).

These symptoms impair the functional capacity and physical well-being of those affected and have been associated with a number of adverse outcomes, including suicidality and premature death (Shalev et al., 2017). See Table 2.1 for diagnostic criteria of ASD and PTSD.

Table 2.1 DIFFERENCES BETWEEN ASD AND PTSD IN ADULTS

	Acute Stress Disorder	*Posttraumatic Stress Disorder*
Criteria	At least nine symptoms regardless of the cluster to which they belong *Note: ASD only includes dissociative amnesia and inability to experience positive emotions as part of altered mood and cognition and does not include reckless and self-destructing behaviors	• At least one intrusion symptom (see above) • At least one avoidance symptom • At least two symptoms of altered mood and cognition • At least two symptoms of marked arousal and reactivity *Note: Derealization is not included in the diagnostic criteria, but can be part of the diagnosis as a concurrent dissociative symptom
Timeline	Between three days and one month	At least one month

TRAUMATIC STRESS IN PATIENTS WITH ADVANCED CANCER

The DSM-5 defines traumatic events as the "exposure to actual or threatened death" (APA, 2013, p. 271). In advanced cancer, this exposure can come in the form of receiving news about the diagnosis, progression, or recurrence of advanced cancer or experiencing distressing symptoms that are reminders of the life-threatening nature of the disease. While traumatic stress symptoms have been well studied in other populations, such as those exposed to physical or sexual assault, the military and police, and first responders to disasters and mass trauma (Shalev et al., 2017), traumatic stress has received much less attention in those with cancer or other life-threatening diseases. The paucity of research examining traumatic stress symptoms in cancer is partly due to the inherent difficulty of recruiting patients into studies at the time of diagnosis, progression, or exacerbation of their illness. At these moments, patients are typically struggling to manage their distress while attempting to navigate a complex health system and make important treatment decisions that have life or death implications. Discussing and retaining unfamiliar medical information can be challenging on its own. One patient in this circumstance said, "I find it very challenging to understand exactly what the doctors are trying to tell me. . . Maybe I can't hear them properly in my absolute panic over what they're saying." During such highly distressing times, participation in research studies is the least important priority for most patients. At the same time, professional understanding of the nature and severity of this experience of trauma is essential to alleviate it.

We have been able to examine the experience of trauma following the diagnosis of acute leukemia, which can be regarded as a prototype for the traumatic stress that is associated with the onset, recurrence, or progression of other life-threatening cancers. Acute leukemia is characterized by an acute onset with immediate threat to life, physical suffering, and the need for urgent hospitalization for the initiation of induction chemotherapy (Rodin et al., 2018; Zimmermann et al., 2013). We have found that clinically significant traumatic stress symptoms occur in a substantial number of patients (Rodin et al., 2013; Zimmermann et al., 2013). In a longitudinal study of over 350 adults newly diagnosed or recently relapsed with acute leukemia, one third reported traumatic stress symptoms that met criteria for threshold or subthreshold ASD, and these symptoms persisted or recurred in more than half of these patients (Rodin et al., 2018). Similar rates of traumatic stress in individuals with newly diagnosed acute leukemia have been reported by others (Jia et al., 2015). These rates are comparable to or higher than those reported following physical assaults or accidents (Kessler et al., 1995). Further, the symptoms of traumatic stress in advanced cancer may be less likely to resolve spontaneously due to the persistent nature of the psychological and physical trauma.

Traumatic stress occurring in the context of cancer is unique in several important ways (Gurevich et al., 2002). Whereas the trauma of physical or sexual assaults or other physical injury is triggered by external events, that related to cancer is linked to events occurring within the body. This internal origin may affect the perception and meaning of the threat and its perceived inescapability (Gurevich et al., 2002). Further, while an assault or accident may be a singular event, the trauma of cancer and its treatment may be chronic and repetitive. It may begin with symptoms that are worrisome and continue with communications about the diagnosis, recurrence, progression, or prognosis of the disease. The ongoing physical suffering related to cancer and/or its treatment, the threat of impending mortality, and the alterations in bodily function or appearance all may represent subsequent traumatic threats. As one CALM participant put it, "There's fear, always. Sometimes you're not even aware of it."

The fear of death and dying, triggered by the diagnosis or progression of advanced disease, constitutes the core component of the initial posttraumatic response. However, patients may not be able to reflect on their fears at this time and may focus instead on more immediate and less threatening practical and treatment-related concerns. In qualitative interviews conducted in the context of our longitudinal study, participants discussed the initial shock of receiving the diagnosis of acute leukemia, often delivered in settings that did not allow for the provision of emotional support and that were focused primarily on the biomedical management of the disease (Nissim et al., 2013). In the early treatment phase, patients tended to surrender control to the medical team, to focus on day-to-day tasks to avoid thoughts about the future, and to choose to receive only a limited amount of information to avoid becoming overwhelmed. As one patient said, "I knew I had to go in for treatment. I didn't want to think about it. I just wanted the hospital to take care of it. I just thought, 'I don't want to know about the numbers and the percentages 'cause it's not going to help me.'"

The reluctance of patients to reflect on future-related fears at this time was related to their high levels of anxiety and their inability to quickly integrate the rapid and dramatic transformation of their lives. Indeed, it may only be later in the disease trajectory that fears about suffering, worries about being a burden to others or about dying and death, and concerns about leaving others behind emerge (Adelbratt & Strang, 2000; Coyle,

2006; Grumann & Spiegel, 2003; Lehto & Stein, 2009; Neel et al., 2015; Smith et al., 1983; Vehling et al., 2017). As one participant noted, "I'm afraid of leaving everybody that I love behind. . . I worry about their well-being." This participant's fear resulted in a frenetic attempt to prepare her family "for the worst": "If I'm dying, my kids need to know where to find their summer hats and sunscreen and so I literally have, in an absolute panic, gone through every cupboard, painted rooms, kept myself super busy in this absolute panic to have things ready in case I do die."

IMPACT ON PRIMARY CAREGIVERS

The diagnosis of cancer is at least as distressing an event for caregivers as it is for patients (Braun et al., 2007; Wadhwa et al., 2013). Traumatic stress symptoms may be as common in caregivers of patients with cancer as they are in patients themselves (Moschopoulou et al., 2018). Moreover, family caregivers of patients with advanced disease may experience a drastic change in their role (Nijboer et al., 1999), progressively becoming the primary source of practical, social, and emotional support for patients (Nijboer et al., 1998; Zabora et al., 1992).

The burden of caregiving has been heightened for many caregivers in recent years because of the shift in the delivery of healthcare from inpatient to outpatient settings. Caregivers are often now implicitly expected to assume a primary role in the delivery of direct patient care, including the administration of medications and the management of physical symptoms, while also maintaining other responsibilities, such as employment or care for other dependents (Mohammed et al., 2018). These burdens fall disproportionately on women (Schrank et al., 2016). Caregivers may also experience distressing thoughts of losing their loved one and witnessing her or his suffering. Primary caregivers are consequently at increased risk of becoming medically ill themselves and of experiencing severe psychological distress, including symptoms of depression, anxiety, and demoralization, compared to similar individuals in the general population (Götze et al., 2018; Mohammed et al., 2018; Williams et al., 2014).

In a study currently being conducted at the Princess Margaret Cancer Centre, primary caregivers of individuals newly diagnosed with acute leukemia are invited to participate in in-depth interviews within the first month after their loved one's diagnosis (Malfitano et al., 2020). Preliminary analyses of these interviews have confirmed that caregivers' distress is intimately connected to and in some respects parallels the experience of the patient (Nissim et al., 2013). Prior to the diagnosis, caregivers report fears related to the uncertain future and possibility of bad outcomes. After the diagnosis, they report a rapid reduction in distress, with an adaptive dissociation from difficult emotions and a focus on short-term milestones and practical tasks. Their distress fluctuates in relation to the patient's health status—only when patients achieve remission and prepare for discharge do caregivers begin to reflect on the long-term impact of the illness, anticipate adjustments, and prepare to grieve losses (Malfitano et al., 2020).

TERROR MANAGEMENT THEORY

Terror management theory is a framework that delineates the personal resources that protect individuals from death anxiety. This framework, which has been extensively studied in healthy populations (Burke et al., 2010), highlights three psychological pillars that serve to protect individuals from the fear of death. These are self-esteem, the sense of meaning in life, and attachment security. Individuals who hold positive beliefs about themselves, find meaning in life, and can create and make use of social support are better able to cope with death anxiety. In most patients with advanced cancer, awareness of a shortened life is inevitable (Cox et al., 2012; Little & Sayers, 2004), and terror management mechanisms therefore become relevant (Portalupi et al., 2016). In support of this, we have found in our research that attachment security, a sense of meaning, and self-esteem protected patients with advanced disease from distress near the end of life (Rodin et al., 2009; also see Chapter 3 of this volume). This evidence has informed CALM, in which there is focused attention on the development of a strong therapeutic relationship that supports attachment security, the sense of meaning, and self-esteem.

THE ROLE OF CALM

Although relief of distress is one of the most important goals of palliative and cancer care, symptoms of traumatic stress and death anxiety have not been routinely measured in either clinical care or clinical trials. Since specialized psychosocial care is often not integrated into the routine care of patients with life-threatening cancer, those who are most in need often do not receive it. Psychotherapeutic approaches such as CALM may be a unique opportunity for patients with advanced cancer to process or manage their fears without becoming overwhelmed or emotionally numb. CALM clinicians pay meticulous attention to fluctuations in the emotional state of the patient and aim to help patients sustain emotional intensity within a range that is tolerable. CALM was developed as both an individual and a couple-based therapy, based on an understanding that illness affects the entire family unit (Edwards & Clarke, 2004; Lewis, 1993) and that patients and their partners represent a "system of mutual influence" (Lo et al., 2013).

CONCLUSION

Intense anxiety, which may meet criteria for ASD or PTSD, is common following the diagnosis of a life-threatening cancer and at subsequent points in the disease trajectory. Death anxiety is the prototypical fear at this time, and terror management theory has helped to delineate the personal resources that individuals require to manage this fear. Although CALM aims to support self-reflection, modulating the intensity of emotions is necessary for self-reflection to occur. The attachment security provided by the therapeutic relationship in CALM may be one of the most important features of CALM therapy in supporting affect regulation, although specific anxiety management techniques may also be required. The successful management of acute traumatic states following diagnosis may allow for reflection on the meaning of the experience at a later point in time and may build confidence in both patients and caregivers in their ability to manage the trauma that inevitably occurs with disease progression. Developing this confidence may be an essential process for so-called posttraumatic growth to occur (see Chapter 8 of this volume).

REFERENCES

Adelbratt, S., & Strang, P. (2000). Death anxiety in brain tumour patients and their spouses. *Palliative Medicine, 14*(6), 499–507.

American Psychiatric Association. (2013). *Diagnostic and statistical manual of mental disorders.* Fifth edition. (DSM-5). American Psychiatric Publishing.

Braun, M., Mikulincer, M., Rydall, A., Walsh, A., & Rodin, G. (2007). Hidden morbidity in cancer: Spouse caregivers. *Journal of Clinical Oncology, 25*(30), 4829–4834.

Burke, B. L., Martens, A., & Faucher, E. H. (2010). Two decades of terror management theory: A meta-analysis of mortality salience research. *Personality and Social Psychology Review, 14*(2), 155–195.

Cox, C. R., Reid-Arndt, S. A., Arndt, J., & Moser, R. P. (2012). Considering the unspoken: The role of death cognition in quality of life among women with and without breast cancer. *Journal of Psychosocial Oncology, 30*(1), 128–139.

Coyle, N. (2006). The hard work of living in the face of death. *Journal of Pain and Symptom Management, 32*(3), 266–274.

Edwards, B., & Clarke, V. (2004). The psychological impact of a cancer diagnosis on families: The influence of family functioning and patients' illness characteristics on depression and anxiety. *Psycho-Oncology, 13*(8), 562–576.

Götze, H., Brähler, E., Gansera, L., Schnabel, A., Gottschalk-Fleischer, A., & Köhler, N. (2018). Anxiety, depression and quality of life in family caregivers of palliative cancer patients during home care and after the patient's death. *European Journal of Cancer Care, 27*(2), e12606. doi: 10.1111/ecc.12606.

Grumann, M. M., & Spiegel, D. (2003). Living in the face of death: Interviews with 12 terminally ill women on home hospice care. *Palliative & Supportive Care, 1*(1), 23–32.

Gurevich, M., Devins, G. M., & Rodin, G. M. (2002). Stress response syndromes and cancer: Conceptual and assessment issues. *Psychosomatics, 43*(4), 259–281.

Jia, M., Li, J., Chen, C., & Cao, F. (2015). Post-traumatic stress disorder symptoms in family caregivers of adult patients with acute leukemia from a dyadic perspective. *Psycho-Oncology, 24*(12), 1754–1760.

Kessler, R. C., Sonnega, A., Bromet, E., Hughes, M., & Nelson, C. B. (1995). Posttraumatic stress disorder in the National Comorbidity Survey. *Archives of General Psychiatry, 52* (12), 1048–1060.

Lehto, R. H., & Stein, K. F. (2009). Death anxiety: An analysis of an evolving concept. *Research and Theory for Nursing Practice, 23*(1), 23–41.

Lewis, F. M. (1993). Psychosocial transitions and the family's work in adjusting to cancer. *Seminars in Oncology Nursing, 9*(2), 127–129.

Little, M., & Sayers, E. J. (2004). The skull beneath the skin: Cancer survival and awareness of death. *Psycho-Oncology, 13*(3), 190–198.

Lo, C., Hales, S., Braun, M., Rydall, A. C., Zimmermann, C., & Rodin, G. (2013). Couples facing advanced cancer: Examination of an interdependent relational system. *Psycho-Oncology, 22*(10), 2283–2290.

Malfitano, C., Caruso, R., Patterson, A., Rydall, A., Nissim, R., Zimmermann, C., & Rodin, G. Zimmermann, C., & Rodin, G. (2020). *Distress in family caregivers of individuals with newly diagnosed acute leukemia.* Paper presented at the 10th International Seminar of the European Palliative Care Research Centre (PRC), in collaboration with the Norwegian Cancer Society, December 3, 2020.

Mohammed, S., Swami, N., Pope, A., Rodin, G., Hannon, B., Nissim, R., Hales, S., & Zimmermann, C. (2018). "I didn't want to be in charge and yet I was": Bereaved caregivers' accounts of providing home care for family members with advanced cancer. *Psycho-Oncology, 27*(4), 1229–1236.

Moschopoulou, E., Hutchison, I., Bhui, K., & Korszun, A. (2018). Post-traumatic stress in head and neck cancer survivors and their partners. *Supportive Care in Cancer, 26* (9), 3003–3011.

Neel, C., Lo, C., Rydall, A., Hales, S., & Rodin, G. (2015). Determinants of death anxiety in patients with advanced cancer. *BMJ Supportive & Palliative Care, 5*(4), 373–380.

Nijboer, C., Tempelaar, R., Sanderman, R., Triemstra, M., Spruijt, R. J., & van den Bos, G. A. (1998). Cancer and caregiving: the impact on the caregiver's health. *Psycho-Oncology, 7*(1), 3–13.

Nijboer, C., Triemstra, M., Tempelaar, R., Sanderman, R., & van den Bos, G. A. (1999). Determinants of caregiving experiences and mental health of partners of cancer patients. *Cancer, 86*(4), 577–588.

Nissim, R., Zimmermann, C., Minden, M., Rydall, A., Yuen, D., Mischitelle, A., Gagliese, L., Schimmer, A., & Rodin, G. (2013). Abducted by the illness: A qualitative study of traumatic stress in individuals with acute leukemia. *Leukemia Research, 37*(5), 496–502.

Portalupi, L. B., Matlock, D. D., Pyszczynski, T. A., & Allen, L. A. (2016). Evidence for terror management theory in patients with chronic progressive illness near the end of life: A systematic review. *Journal of Cardiac Failure, 22*(8), Supplement, S105.

Rodin, G., Deckert, A., Tong, E., Le, L. W., Rydall, A., Schimmer, A., Marmar, C. R., Lo, C., & Zimmermann, C. (2018). Traumatic stress in patients with acute leukemia: A prospective cohort study. *Psycho-Oncology, 27*(2), 515–523.

Rodin, G., Lo, C., Mikulincer, M., Donner, A., Gagliese, L., & Zimmermann, C. (2009). Pathways to distress: The multiple determinants of depression, hopelessness, and the desire for hastened death in metastatic cancer patients. *Social Science & Medicine, 68*(3), 562–569.

Rodin, G., Yuen, D., Mischitelle, A., Minden, M. D., Brandwein, J., Schimmer, A., Marmar, C., Gagliese, L., Lo, C., Rydall, A., & Zimmermann, C. (2013). Traumatic stress in acute leukemia. *Psycho-Oncology, 22*(2), 299–307.

Schrank, B., Ebert-Vogel, A., Amering, M., Masel, E. K., Neubauer, M., Watzke, H., Zehetmayer, S., & Schur, S. (2016). Gender differences in caregiver burden and its determinants in family members of terminally ill cancer patients. *Psycho-Oncology, 25*(7), 808–814.

Shalev, A., Liberzon, I., & Marmar, C. (2017). Post-traumatic stress disorder. *New England Journal of Medicine, 376*(25), 2459–2469.

Smith, D. K., Nehemkis, A. M., & Charter, R. A. (1983–1984). Fear of death, death attitudes, and religious conviction in the terminally ill. *International Journal of Psychiatry in Medicine, 13*(3), 221–232.

Vehling, S., Malfitano, C., Shnall, J., Watt, S., Panday, T., Chiu, A., Rydall, A., Zimmermann, C., Hales, S., Rodin, G., & Lo, C. (2017). A concept map of death-related anxieties in patients with advanced cancer. *BMJ Supportive & Palliative Care, 7*(4), 427–434.

Wadhwa, D., Burman, D., Swami, N., Rodin, G., Lo, C., & Zimmermann, C. (2013). Quality of life and mental health in caregivers of outpatients with advanced cancer. *Psycho-Oncology, 22*(2), 403–410.

Williams, A. M., Wang, L., & Kitchen, P. (2014). Differential impacts of care-giving across three caregiver groups in Canada: End-of-life care, long-term care and short-term care. *Health & Social Care in the Community, 22*(2), 187–196.

Zabora, J. R., Smith, E. D., Baker, F., Wingard, J. R., & Curbow, B. (1992). The family: The other side of bone marrow transplantation. *Journal of Psychosocial Oncology, 10*(1), 35–46.

Zimmermann, C., Yuen, D., Mischitelle, A., Minden, M. D., Brandwein, J. M., Schimmer, A., Gagliese, L., Lo, C., Rydall, A., & Rodin, G. (2013). Symptom burden and supportive care in patients with acute leukemia. *Leukemia Research, 37*(7), 731–736.

CHAPTER 3

One Thousand Lives

The Work That Influenced CALM

We are in the middle of wreckage, of incredible destruction, and we are also surrounded by this phenomenal natural burst of life.

—Will to Live study participant

INTRODUCTION

Managing Cancer and Living Meaningfully (CALM) builds upon the foundational work of earlier researchers and upon our own clinical experience and research over the past two decades with more than 1,000 patients with advanced cancer and as many or more bereaved caregivers. In this chapter, we will describe how this work led to the development of CALM, focusing in particular on two of our major research projects: The Will to Live (WTL) study and the Quality of Dying and Death (QODD) study.

EARLY GROUNDBREAKING RESEARCH

The collective works of pioneers such as Kübler-Ross (1969), Glaser and Strauss (1965), and Pattison (1977) have had a dramatic effect on our understanding of the psychological impact of advanced disease. In *On Death and Dying*, Kübler-Ross suggested that the psychological response to a diagnosis of a fatal illness is most often a sequential process, beginning with denial and followed by anger, bargaining, depression, and ultimately with acceptance. Denial was viewed as a necessary emotional buffer of the impact of the initial shocking news. Anger and bargaining were postulated to follow as short-lived reactions to the understanding that death is near. Depression was then said to set in when the individual began to mourn the losses associated with the illness, which was necessary before a stage of peaceful acceptance could be reached. A lack of progression through these stages was considered to reflect adaptive failure.

Kübler-Ross's (1969) five-stage model quickly became the main paradigm in the field (Corr et al., 1999; Steinhauser, 2005), although it was also criticized (Copp, 1998; Côté & Pepler, 2005; Morse, 2000; Zimmermann, 2004). In particular, the unidirectional movement from denial to acceptance postulated by Kübler-Ross was challenged. Weisman (1972) and Pattison (1977) both suggested that denial and acceptance may fluctuate throughout the illness, and Weisman further posited that denial not only serves to diminish the threat of death but also to avoid burdening others, such as family members or healthcare providers. Nevertheless, Kübler-Ross's work continues to have a profound impact on the way that psychological response to fatal illness is conceptualized in Western society.

During the period in which Kübler-Ross (1969) conducted her work, Glaser and Strauss (1965, 1968) were investigating the social organization of dying in American hospitals. They coined the term "the dying trajectory" to denote that dying is a process, not an event, and that its duration and shape determines how it is managed by hospital staff (Glaser & Strauss, 1968, p. 5). In this vein, Pattison (1977; 1978, p. 49) referred to the living–dying interval as the duration of time between the "crisis of knowledge of death" and the actual point of death. Pattison suggested that there are specific clinical tasks that must be performed at each phase of the living–dying interval. In the acute crisis phase, healthcare professionals are called upon to support patients with the stress of diagnosis. The chronic living–dying phase—a phase that has become more common in recent years due to advances in cancer treatment that have prolonged survival—is focused on resolving fears of dying and on mourning the multiple losses associated with the prospect of death. The task for healthcare professionals in the final terminal phase involves helping patients reach a comfortable death.

Kübler-Ross (1969), Glaser and Strauss (1965), and Pattison (1977, 1978) opened the field of death and dying to investigation, inspiring others to conduct research on the psychosocial needs of individuals with advanced disease and stimulating changes in how care is delivered to these individuals. However, their views on adjustment to advanced disease were primarily derived from the professional perspective of the health-care provider, rather than from that of the ill individual. They proposed that professionals could shift reactions deemed "pathological" to ones considered more adaptive and appropriate (Corr et al., 1999). This well-intentioned view was consistent with the more hierarchical view of the physician–patient relationship that was prevalent at that time.

The role of patients in their healthcare began to shift dramatically in the last part of the 20th century, when their rights to autonomy and self-determination were legitimized and legalized in many societies (Charles et al., 1999). This gave rise to more patient-centered models of care, some of which detailed a set of physical, psychological, spiritual, and social tasks for patients to accomplish in the final weeks of life (Byock, 1997; Corr, 1992; Doka, 1993). Completion of these tasks was regarded as a sign of successful coping with death and dying, allowing for growth, a sense of completion near the end of life, and preparedness for death. These task-based models were consistent with those developed for the successful resolution of bereavement and grief (Corr et al., 1999). However, they lacked empirical support (Copp, 1998) and were subsequently replaced by the view that bereavement is an active process involving a duality between loss and restoration (Stroebe et al., 1998). Such dualistic models regarding the experience of fatal illness were uncommon at that time.

Much of the early research on adjustment to advanced disease consisted of cross-sectional studies that assessed quality of life and suffering at the end of life (Steinhauser, 2005). This research was often limited by the lack of appropriate and validated measures (Steinhauser et al., 2002) and by the lack of attention to the earlier stages of advanced disease. While it provided valuable information on the experience of individuals at the end of life (Copp, 1998), patients with cancer and other medical conditions were spending longer periods of time living with their disease before death (Good et al., 2004; Lynn, 2005). They more often came to enjoy plateaus in disease progression, with relatively good functioning for months after diagnosis (Diaz-Rubio, 2004; Lunney et al., 2003; Stinnett et al., 2007). As this living–dying interval (Pattison, 1977) became more prolonged, the most pressing question for those diagnosed with advanced cancer became how to live well, rather than simply how to die well (Walter, 2003). However, there had been little research conducted, particularly longitudinal studies, to capture this prolonged experience of living with advanced cancer (e.g., George, 2002; Hays, 2003; Lynn, 2005; Seale, 2000; Steinhauser, 2005). Cross-sectional studies provided important information but could not capture the experience of patients with advanced disease from the time of diagnosis to the end of life.

We undertook the WTL and the QODD projects to understand the experience of advanced cancer through the eyes of patients and their caregivers as it unfolded over time. Over more than five years, we recruited over 700 patients from outpatient clinics at the Princess Margaret Cancer Centre, a large comprehensive cancer center in Toronto, Canada, to participate in the longitudinal WTL study. Participants had a confirmed diagnosis of Stage IV (metastatic) gastrointestinal or Stage IIIA, IIIB, or IV (recurrent or metastatic) lung cancer. Of those recruited into this study, we followed more than 400 to the end of life, using self-report measures to assess their psychological well-being. A subset of participants was invited to participate in qualitative interviews, with the data analyzed using the grounded theory method (Glaser & Strauss, 1967, subsequently modified for psychological inquiry by Rennie et al., 1988).

We found that the lived experience of advanced cancer was often highly distressing (Lo et al., 2010). More than one third of our sample reported at least mild depressive symptoms at some point over the course of their illness, and half of these individuals reported moderate to severe depression. To what extent distress of this kind occurred or persisted in specific individuals depended on a complex interplay of multiple risk and protective factors (Rodin et al., 2009). Psychological factors, such as self-esteem, attachment security, and spiritual well-being—the pillars of terror management theory (see Chapter 2 of this volume)—protected against depression, while physical symptom burden greatly increased its risk (see Figure 3.1). Hopelessness, a construct distinct from but related to depression, was triggered by existential concerns about meaning, peace, and faith.

We found curvilinear growth in depressive symptoms as individuals approached the end of life (Lo et al., 2010; see Figure 3.2). In fact, the proportion of participants with significant depression in the final three months of life was triple that found in individuals who were furthest from death. This increase in distress in the final months of life seemed due both to the increase in disease burden and to the proximity to death (Lo et al., 2010). However, in contrast to the more linear model of Kübler-Ross (1969), this distress fluctuated over the course of the illness, suggesting an ongoing, dynamic adaptation to the multiple losses and challenges that occurred over the course of the disease. We came to believe that these challenges—particularly those related to symptom burden and existential distress—would impair the quality of life and quality of dying and death in patients with advanced cancer unless proactively addressed. These discoveries suggested that interventions were needed to relieve physical,

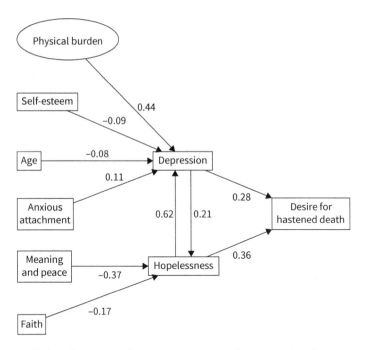

Figure 3.1. Risk and protective factors contributing to depression, hopelessness, and the desire for death

Reprinted from Rodin, G., Lo, C., Mikulincer, M., Donner, A., Gagliese, L., & Zimmermann, C. (2009). Pathways to distress: The multiple determinants of depression, hopelessness, and the desire for hastened death in metastatic cancer patients. *Social Science & Medicine, 68*(3); 562–569, with permission from Elsevier.

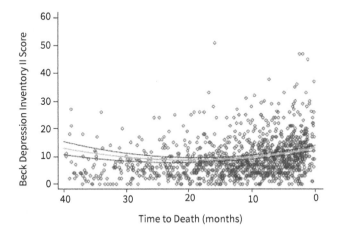

Figure 3.2. Curvilinear growth of depression as a reflect of time to death

Lo, C., Zimmermann, C., Rydall, A., Walsh, A., Jones, J. M., Moore, M. J., Shepherd, F. A., Gagliese, L., & Rodin, G. (2010). Longitudinal study of depressive symptoms in patients with metastatic gastrointestinal and lung cancer. *Journal of Clinical Oncology, 28*(18), 3084–3089. Reprinted with permission. © (2010) American Society of Clinical Oncology. All rights reserved.

psychological, and spiritual distress and provided an empirical impetus to the development of CALM.

Our quantitative research elucidated the prevalence and nature of distress in advanced cancer, but our qualitative studies generated a deeper understanding of the prolonged experience of advanced disease. Using the grounded theory method, we organized our understanding by a core category of "Striving to Grow in the Land of the Living/Dying," and second-level categories of "The Land of the Living/Dying" and "Striving to Grow" (Nissim et al., 2012). The first equated the new circumstances of advanced cancer to being placed in an unfamiliar and dangerous land, which was terra incognita. The second depicted the wish to cling to life and to adapt to and navigate this new land. Together, these categories comprised a synthesis between the inevitable and the possible, with the Striving to Grow continuously informed by the bewildering array of mental, spiritual, physical, and social injuries imposed by the illness. These categories are expanded upon next.

The Land of the Living/Dying

The Land of the Living/Dying likens the experience of being diagnosed with advanced cancer to being placed in an indeterminate state between living and dying. It is akin to being deported from a familiar land, the Land of the Living, to an unfamiliar place, where the roadmaps of the previous land do not apply. As one participant said, "As soon as I wake up . . . the realization hits me that I have cancer now, that I have this terminal disease, and that today is different than all the other days I've been used to all my life." Participants often highlighted the difference between the experience of advanced cancer and that of previous health problems that were either resolvable or not life-threatening. As one participant explained,

> It is one thing to go in and say, 'Okay, I am going to put up with this chemo for six months and then my chances are really good, that's going to be it.' You only have that time period; you can invest that much energy into that time period. But if you are terminal you don't know what the hell is going on, you just kind of cross your fingers and go into it.

Transfer to the new land was regarded by patients as more of a process than an event. Most commonly, receiving the news of the diagnosis was followed by weeks of trying to understand and verify this new territory and determine whether the "death sentence" could be appealed. It took some time for participants to believe that they were permanently in a new land. Enrollment in a clinical trial immediately after diagnosis often postponed the feeling of being in the Living/Dying Land. Some participants only felt permanently domiciled there when repeated clinical trials did not eradicate the cancer. As one noted, "Only then . . . I knew where I stood, I really understood the truth of this whole thing." When the diagnosis was made in the context of a sudden and critical medical event, the full experience of being in a new land was delayed until the immediate crisis was resolved. Five categories of experience that were identified in the Land of the Living/Dying are described next:

1. *The specter of finitude.* The finitude of life was palpable and a constant specter for many participants. They reported feeling an "unnatural" sense of being "always on the verge of dying," using metaphors such as "living on death row" or "living with a time bomb." As one said, "Of course any man has to die. But a healthy person does not need to think about it. It may happen 30, 40, or 50 years later. You can live happily. But for us—we can never not think about death." This became evident when participants were asked about renewing a club membership, about holiday plans, and even about another research interview in upcoming months. The specter of finitude was felt as a constant, heavy burden that brought sadness and grief about being excluded from further participation in the experience of life. It was present in older individuals but was most overpowering for those who were raising young children. These participants grieved not only the loss of their future, but its impact on the future of their children.

2. *Dread of a lingering death.* Being in the Land of the Living/Dying was associated with a new preoccupation for participants, which was the manner in which they would die. Whereas those in the land of the living tend to fear death as an unforeseen and sudden event, those in the Land of the Living/Dying worried that it would be a lingering, undignified, and painful process for themselves and their families that would deprive them of a sense of personhood and meaning. The imagined process of such a death was terrifying and typically much more difficult for participants to accept than death itself. At the time of the study, the dread of a lingering death was fueled by the emerging public debate and media coverage in Canada on assisted dying and by personal experiences of participants with friends or relatives who had died from cancer. Participants recalled memories of the final days of relatives and friends, thinking, "I don't want to be that way."

The dread of a lingering death was heightened when there was a lack of discussion with physicians about the end of life and a focus in clinical encounters on present problems, rather than on future concerns. Participants felt that initiating discussions regarding future scenarios would either be a waste of the oncologist's valuable time, a taboo topic, or would be taken to mean that they did not wish to continue anticancer treatments. However, this lack of discussion about what awaited them made the process of death even more dreaded. The resulting void of knowledge was filled by personal and cultural stereotypes of dying of cancer and heightened their fears about the ability of the medical profession to palliate symptoms at the end of life.

3. *Medical uncertainty.* Although there was certainty in the Land of the Living/Dying that death would occur, there was much uncertainty about when it would take place. Participants often experienced this terrain as a medical no man's land in which new treatment protocols continued to be developed, and individual responses to treatment were impossible to predict. One participant likened consenting to an anticancer treatment to being in "an experiment with one lab rat." Participants also commented on their frustration with the lack of clear medical recommendations and with repeatedly hearing that "every cancer is different." They often found medical uncertainty to be more terrifying than the certainty of death. As one said, "We all know we are going to die so the actual thought of death is not the scary part. What is scary is them telling you that you are going to die and we are not sure if it is going to be in three months or a year; we are not sure how painful it is going to be, sometimes it is and sometimes it's not."

4. *Physical suffering.* Physical suffering was common, with participants reporting an average of eight physical symptoms related to their cancer, and contributed to a sense of unfamiliarity with their bodily experience. Sensations such as pain and fatigue that may have been previously experienced as benign now had more ominous implications. As one said, "The pain is telling me that I'm dying. It's telling me it's winning this time. Because it's a really nasty pain. . . It's a different kind of pain. It speaks so directly to you. It says, 'I've gotcha.'" There were also frightening new physical symptoms, such as loss of coordination, breathing problems, or difficulty swallowing. Physical suffering in the Land of the Living/Dying fluctuated, contributing to a "roller-coaster feeling." Periods of extreme physical suffering brought more uncertainty, fear, grief, despair, and a sense of a tightening trap. In contrast, when there were fewer physical challenges, participants experienced a sense of relief that was likened to being in "calm water."

5. *Uninhabited land.* The diagnosis of advanced cancer was uniformly described by participants as causing them to feel stigmatized, marginalized, isolated, and "rejected," or to feel treated as "dead already." The isolation was heightened by the perceived inability of others to understand the unique mental and physical landscape of the Land of the Living/Dying. As one participant noted, "They start saying things like, 'Well, you know, I could get hit by a truck tomorrow crossing the street just as easily.' But it's not the same."

The sense of being in an uninhabited land was amplified by the difficulty of discussing their experience with others. Participants commonly spoke of the challenge of talking with family members and friends about the realities of the new land, because they believed that their loved ones would be uncomfortable with the topic. The participants tended to dodge questions about their experience to protect or avoid burdening family members and friends. The sense of being in an uninhabited land was also attributed by participants to the void in mass media and culture regarding the prolonged experience of living with advanced illness, an experience that defied conventional boundaries of living and dying. In this regard, participants talked about the lack of a cultural script or a "textbook" to follow when in the Land of the Living/Dying and about their failed search to find, as one said, "a set of rules of how you're supposed to act."

Striving to Grow

Being in the Land of the Living/Dying seemed to highlight for many participants the force of life and the power of the will to live. They spoke about a relentless striving, not just to survive, but to live dynamically and to find ways to grow and engage in life regardless of their devastating circumstances. One participant described it as a striving "to do what I can, to the best of my ability, for as long as I'm alive." They said that they were labeled by others as "courageous," but they regarded their Striving to Grow instead as an instinct and the natural thing to do when trapped in a dangerous new land. The following excerpt wonderfully elaborates this paradox, using the metaphor of the germinating fireweed to capture the "burst of life" experienced in the midst of "incredible destruction."

> I was thinking about a trip I took to Europe. It is like a picture in my mind, like a moving film. We saw a church that was burned during the Second World War, the ruins were covered with flowers called fireweed and this flower was

astonishing, very strong color. This flower looks like fire, but this is not why it is called fireweed. The reason it is called fireweed is that it hasn't been seen in London since the great fire in 1607, and they couldn't understand how this weed survived, and germinated again. And it turned out that the seeds are rock hard and it takes a fire to burn the outer shell. The destructive fire is the only way by which the seed can crack open, and moisture can get in, and it germinates again. And the flowers were everywhere and it was the strangest thing. We are in the middle of wreckage, of incredible destruction and we are also surrounded by this phenomenal natural burst of life and it was overpowering, and I'm thinking about it and I realize that it is like a metaphor for my life right at the moment. It is like this thing that happened to me, being diagnosed with cancer, has broken down all the old barriers I had around my life, and my attitude to living.

The Striving to Grow is akin to the concept of posttraumatic growth (see Chapter 8 of this volume), which involves setting new goals and moving to actualize them while grieving lost capabilities and potentialities. Participants identified opportunities that remained available to them or that emerged anew within the changing parameters of their illness. Fulfilling these goals brought meaning, satisfaction, and joy in the time left to live, although despair emerged when all pathways to actualizing their goals appeared to be blocked. These states of despair tended to be transient, and participants tended to remain determined to actualize goals along the illness trajectory, to the extent that this was possible. Overall, they described an oscillation between defining and actualizing goals, then facing despair, and then finding a way to set goals again. This continued until the oscillation was replaced by a final letting go, a capitulation to the final physical collapse in the last days of life.

THE QUALITY OF DYING AND DEATH STUDY

CALM is intended to help patients with advanced disease live meaningfully and face the end of life with peace and equanimity. The extent to which the latter occurs is captured in the multidimensional construct of the "quality of dying and death," which includes physical, psychological, social, spiritual, and existential experiences at the end of life (Hales et al., 2008). However, when we began to develop CALM, we found that there was very little research examining the quality of dying and death of patients with advanced cancer from the perspective of those involved in the process (Goodman, 2011; Heyland et al., 2005). To learn more about this, we initiated a large retrospective study—the first of its kind—to assess the quality of dying and death in a Canadian urban setting.

In the QODD study, we interviewed over 400 bereaved adult caregivers of patients with metastatic cancer six months after the death of their loved one using the QODD questionnaire (Patrick et al., 2001) and measures of psychological well-being. The QODD, in which caregivers act as proxies for the patients, is the most widely used and best-validated instrument to assess the quality of dying and death (Hales et al., 2010). We waited six months after the death of the patient to conduct these interviews so as not to intrude on caregivers during their grieving period, and this delay did not appear to affect caregivers' abilities to recall details of their loved ones' deaths. We were able to examine the quality of dying and death in cancer patients whose deaths occurred in inpatient, outpatient, and home-based palliative care settings. It should be noted that this study was conducted in an urban center in which the large majority of patients had access to early palliative care.

Most bereaved caregivers in our study denied symptoms of depression and hopelessness, and the majority rated their loved ones' deaths as "good" or "almost perfect" (Hales et al., 2014). However, despite the high ratings by the majority of caregivers, physical symptom control and transcendence over death-related concerns were rated as "terrible" to "poor" in 15% and 19% of cases, respectively. The unsatisfactory experience of a substantial minority of patients in these categories made us wonder whether the implementation of CALM earlier in the disease course would have allowed some of these patients to face the end of life with less fear and suffering.

CONCLUSION

Medical progress in prolonging survival in advanced cancer has created a new experience of dying, in which an indeterminate state of living/dying can last for years. This brought a call for research to produce "the language, the categories, and the stories" (Lynn, 2005, p. 14) of those with a prolonged trajectory of dying. The longitudinal research described here helped to illuminate the complexity of the living/dying trajectory and the duality of the experience of advanced cancer—the intensity of the loss and the desire for continued self-actualization that accompanies it. This view challenged earlier explanatory models that emphasized clinical tasks to be accomplished to resolve the stress, fear, and grief of dying (Pattison, 1977) and those postulating a more linear progression of psychological reactions to death (Kübler-Ross, 1969). Our findings suggest that fear and loss can never be fully resolved and oscillate instead with a profound striving to live life as fully as possible. Our findings align with other research in medical populations demonstrating that hope is multidimensional and dynamic and extends far beyond the hope for a cure (Fitzgerald Miller, 2007; Gum & Snyder, 2002; Parse, 1999). The knowledge about the experience of advanced cancer resulting from our work has helped to shape CALM, highlighting the need to help patients face their fears while also engaging in life.

REFERENCES

Byock, I. (1997). *Dying well: The prospect for growth at the end of life*. Riverhead Books.

Charles, C., Gafni, A., & Whelan, T. (1999). Decision-making in the physician–patient encounter: Revisiting the shared treatment decision-making model. *Social Science & Medicine, 49*(5), 651–661.

Copp, G. (1998). A review of current theories of death and dying. *Journal of Advanced Nursing, 28*(2), 382–390.

Corr, C. A. (1992). A task-based approach to coping with dying. *OMEGA-Journal of Death and Dying, 24*(2), 81–94.

Corr, C. A., Doka, K. J., & Kastenbaum, R. (1999). Dying and its interpreters: A review of selected literature and some comments on the state of the field. *OMEGA-Journal of Death and Dying, 39*(4), 239–259.

Côté, J. K., & Pepler, C. (2005). A focus for nursing intervention: Realistic acceptance or helping illusions? *International Journal of Nursing Practice, 11*(1), 39–43.

Diaz-Rubio, E. (2004). New chemotherapeutic advances in pancreatic, colorectal, and gastric cancers. *The Oncologist, 9*(3), 282–294.

Doka, K. J. (1993). *Living with life-threatening illness*. Lexington Books.

Fitzgerald Miller, J. (2007). Hope: A construct central to nursing. *Nursing Forum, 42*(1), 12–19.

George, L. K. (2002). Research design in end-of-life research: State of science. *The Gerontologist, 42*(Suppl. 3), 86–98.

Glaser, B. G., & Strauss, A. L. (1965). *Awareness of dying*. Aldine Transaction.

Glaser, B. G., & Strauss, A. L. (1967). *The discovery of grounded theory: Strategies for qualitative research*. Aldine Transaction.

Glaser, B. G., & Strauss, A. L. (1968). *Time for dying*. Aldine Transaction.

Good, P. D., Cavenagh, J., & Ravenscroft, P. J. (2004). Survival after enrollment in an Australian palliative care program. *Journal of Pain and Symptom Management, 27*(4), 310–315.

Goodman, D. (2011). End-of-life cancer care in Ontario and the United States: Quality by accident or quality by design? *Journal of the National Cancer Institute, 103*(11), 840–841.

Gum, A., & Snyder, C. R. (2002). Coping with terminal illness: The role of hopeful thinking. *Journal of Palliative Medicine, 5*(6), 883–894.

Hales, S., Chiu, A., Husain, A., Braun, M., Rydall, A., Gagliese, L., Zimmermann, C., & Rodin, G. (2014). The quality of dying and death in cancer and its relationship to palliative care and place of death. *Journal of Pain and Symptom Management, 48*(5), 839–851.

Hales, S., Zimmermann, C., & Rodin, G. (2008). The quality of dying and death. *Archives of Internal Medicine, 168*(9), 912–918.

Hales, S., Zimmermann, C., & Rodin, G. (2010). The quality of dying and death: A systematic review of measures. *Palliative Medicine, 24*(2), 127–144.

Hays, J. C. (2003). Busy/dying. *Public Health Nursing, 20*(3), 165–166.

Heyland, D. K., Groll, D., Rocker, G., Dodek, P., Gafni, A., Tranmer, J., Pichora, D., Lazar, N., Kutsogiannis, J., Shortt, S., Lam, M.; Canadian Researchers at the End of Life Network (CARENET). (2005). End-of-life care in acute care hospitals in Canada: A quality finish? *Journal of Palliative Care, 21*(3), 142–150.

Kübler-Ross, E. (1969). *On death and dying*. Tavistock. Publications.

Lo, C., Zimmermann, C., Rydall, A., Walsh, A., Jones, J. M., Moore, M. J., Shepherd, F.A., Gagliese, L., & Rodin, G. (2010). Longitudinal study of depressive symptoms in patients with metastatic gastrointestinal and lung cancer. *Journal of Clinical Oncology, 28*(18), 3084–3089.

Lunney, J. R., Lynn, J., Foley, D. J., Lipson, S., & Guralnik, J. M. (2003). Patterns of functional decline at the end of life. *JAMA, 289*(18), 2387–2392.

Lynn, J. (2005). Living long in fragile health: The new demographics shape end of life care. *Hastings Center Report, 35*(Suppl 6), s14–s18.

Morse, J. M. (2000). Denial is not a qualitative concept. *Qualitative Health Research, 10*(2), 147–148.

Nissim, R., Rennie, D., Fleming, S., Hales, S., Gagliese, L., & Rodin, G. (2012). Goals set in the land of the living/dying: A longitudinal study of patients living with advanced cancer. *Death Studies, 36*(4), 360–390.

Parse, R. R. (1999). *Hope: An international human becoming perspective*. Jones & Bartlett Learning.

Patrick, D. L., Engelberg, R. A., & Curtis, J. R. (2001). Evaluating the quality of dying and death. *Journal of Pain and Symptom Management, 22*(3), 717–726.

Pattison, E. M. (1977). *The experience of dying*. Prentice Hall.

Pattison, E. M. (1978). The living–dying process. In C. A. Garfield (Ed.), *Psychosocial care of the dying patient* (pp. 133–168). McGraw-Hill.

Rennie, D. L., Phillips, J. R., & Quartaro, G. K. (1988). Grounded theory: A promising approach to conceptualization in psychology? *Canadian Psychology/Psychologie Canadienne, 29*(2), 139–150.

Rodin, G., Lo, C., Mikulincer, M., Donner, A., Gagliese, L., & Zimmermann, C. (2009). Pathways to distress: The multiple determinants of depression, hopelessness, and the desire for hastened death in metastatic cancer patients. *Social Science & Medicine, 68*(3), 562–569.

Seale, C. (2000). Changing patterns of death and dying. *Social Science & Medicine, 51*(6), 917–930.

Steinhauser, K. E. (2005). Measuring end-of-life care outcomes prospectively. *Journal of Palliative Medicine, 8*(Suppl. 1), S 30–41.

Steinhauser, K. E., Clipp, E. C., & Tulsky, J. A. (2002). Evolution in measuring the quality of dying. *Journal of Palliative Medicine, 5*(3), 407–414.

Stinnett, S., Williams, L., & Johnson, D. H. (2007). Role of chemotherapy for palliation in the lung cancer patient. *The Journal of Supportive Oncology, 5*(1), 19–24.

Stroebe, M., Schut, H., & Stroebe, W. (1998). Trauma and grief: A comparative analysis. In J. H. Harvey (Ed.), *Perspectives on loss: A sourcebook* (pp. 81–96). Brunner/Mazel.

Walter, T. (2003). Historical and cultural variants on the good death. *BMJ, 327*(7408), 218–220.

Weisman, A. D. (1972). *On dying and denying: A psychiatric study of terminality.* Behavioural Publications.

Zimmermann, C. (2004). Denial of impending death: A discourse analysis of the palliative care literature. *Social Science & Medicine, 59*(8), 1769–1780.

CHAPTER 4
Attachment Security

CALM has given me space and time that I just haven't had to talk about things that are really important. It feels like what a home might mean for a person who has been homeless.
            —CALM participant

INTRODUCTION

Connection to others is a fundamental human need that sustains psychological well-being and the will to live (Khan et al., 2010). Attachment security refers to the internal sense of this connection and the willingness and capacity to seek and accept emotional support from others. Attachment theory is a powerful explanatory framework for understanding the relational needs of patients and families facing the crisis of a serious or life-threatening illness. It is relevant to personal and family relationships, to relationships with healthcare providers, and to relationships with others who are experienced as supportive in the relief of distress. The Managing Cancer and Living Meaningfully (CALM) therapist can support attachment security in patients and play an important role in helping them renegotiate their attachment relationships in light of the heightened emotional distress and diminished capacity for autonomy that occur with advanced disease. This chapter will provide background on attachment security and its application to CALM therapy.

John Bowlby was a psychiatrist and psychoanalyst who first applied the construct of attachment security to the understanding of human psychological development and the psychotherapeutic process. His interest in the subject began in the mid-20th century with his clinical work in a home for maladjusted boys separated from their mothers, and he began to outline his theory of attachment in his three-volume book, *Attachment and Loss* (Bowlby, 1969, 1973, 1980). Bowlby emphasized the fundamental importance of attachment relationships in psychological development and highlighted the survival value of behavioral systems that keep us in close proximity to caregivers, particularly in times of heightened danger. He outlined general attachment tendencies that could be described as secure or insecure, depending on the child's expectation of caregiver availability and their view of themselves as acceptable or unacceptable in the eyes of the attachment figure.

Bowlby and colleagues began their work by examining relationships between children and mothers, but attachment theory was later applied to a wide range of adult relationships. These have included relationships with romantic partners (Kunce & Shaver, 1994) and those between patients and their healthcare providers (Maunder & Hunter, 2016). Attachment security in adults can be assessed with semi-structured interviews such as the Adult Attachment Interview (George et al., 1996) or with self-report questionnaires, such as the Experiences in Close Relationships Inventory (ECR; Brennan et al., 1998; Fraley et al., 2000). The latter assesses anxious and avoidant attachment, two main dimensions of attachment security. Anxious attachment refers to the tendency to feel unable to cope and to fear that necessary support will not be available; avoidant attachment refers to the tendency to be self-reliant and to minimize expressions of distress (Bowlby, 1980).

The original ECR (Brennan et al., 1998) and its revised versions (Fraley et al., 2000) are 36-item self-report measures that assess attachment tendencies in romantic relationships. However, because the experience of attachment security can be derived from many others, including healthcare providers, and because a briefer measure is more feasible for patients with advanced disease to complete, we created a modified, briefer 16-item measure referred to as the ECR-M16 (Lo et al., 2009). The ECR-M16 assesses attachment security more generally in relationships with supportive others. We have demonstrated the reliability and validity of this measure (Lo et al., 2009) and have utilized it extensively in our research program and in the clinical application of CALM (see Chapter 10 of this volume).

Bowlby (1969) proposed that attachment security is a fundamental human need "from the cradle to the grave" (Bowlby, 1969, p. 208). The attachment system supports psychological and physical well-being and is activated in response to threat. In advanced disease, this may include fears of pain or other physical suffering, dependency, loss of control, or the threat of dying and death. When it is activated, proximity to caregivers or other attachment figures is sought to relieve distress and restore emotional equilibrium. Those with greater attachment security may be better able to seek and accept practical and emotional assistance to relieve distress. The benefit of attachment security in protecting from the terror of death anxiety has been highlighted in the theoretical framework of terror management theory (TMT; Greenberg, 2012; see Chapter 2 of this volume).

TMT has been largely studied and validated in healthy populations in which death anxiety is experimentally simulated or evoked (Burke et al., 2010). Our group has extended research on TMT by examining the protective effect of attachment security in patients with advanced disease who face the literal threat of death. In the Will to Live study (see Chapter 3 of this volume), we demonstrated that attachment security protects patients with advanced disease from depression as their physical symptom burden grows (Rodin et al., 2007). Those with less attachment security may be in "double jeopardy," because they not only lack confidence or trust in support from others, but they are also less likely to have or to make appropriate use of supportive relationships. Early developmental experiences play an important role in the formation of attachment security, but longitudinal studies have shown that attachment security may grow or deteriorate over time, depending on the nature and quality of personal relationships (McConnell & Moss, 2011).

Individuals with greater attachment security have a flexibility in relationships that allows them to seek help from others when it is needed and to experience relief of distress. The anxiously attached tend to be worried about the availability of support and to lack confidence in their ability to manage the challenges of their disease; those who are more avoidantly attached tend to minimize distress and the need for support (Tan et al., 2005). Research with patients with advanced cancer has shown that both anxious and avoidant attachment styles are associated with less perceived emotional support and greater distress (Hunter et al., 2006). Those with a disorganized attachment style lack a coherent and consistent approach to attachment relationships—described as "fright without solutions"—and may find it difficult to find relief from relationships with others (Main, 1995).

Not only may attachment theory explain differences in support-seeking and distress at the end of life, but it may also shape attitudes toward the end of life and palliative care. Attachment-related themes that emerge at the end of life include those related to autonomy and control, privacy boundaries, social support, the tenor of care, and the sense of being a burden to others (Chochinov et al., 2002). Those with an avoidant attachment style are more likely to experience the loss of dignity with advanced disease (Tan et al., 2005). It has been reported that requests for medical assistance in dying are related to an avoidant attachment style, the desire to maintain a sense of personal control, and the wish to avoid anticipated dependency and loss of autonomy (Ganzini et al., 2009). We have wondered to what extent psychotherapeutic interventions, such as CALM, can ameliorate or prevent this outcome.

ATTACHMENT AND CAREGIVING IN ADVANCED DISEASE

Caregivers supporting a loved one with a life-threatening illness are called upon to aid in navigation of the healthcare system, access information, liaise with medical personnel, and provide transportation, economic aid, and physical and emotional support for patients. In addition to the stresses of providing care, the threat of their loved one's death may require the caregiver to prepare to lose an important attachment figure of their own. The healthcare system in all parts of the world depends on informal caregivers to support patients with advanced cancer, although there has been insufficient attention to their needs (Glajchen, 2004; Grunfeld et al., 2004).

Caregivers of those with advanced disease who deeply care about the needs and suffering of their loved one may also feel the need to distance themselves to prepare for a life ahead without their partner (Evans, 1994; Johansson & Grimby, 2012; Parkes, 1996). Research has shown that those who are more securely attached have more capacity for effective caregiving. Individuals who are more avoidantly attached are less likely to provide care or tend to provide care that is insensitive and controlling. The caregiving of those who are anxiously attached tends to be compulsively driven by the needs and anxieties of the caregiver rather than by those of the patient (Kunce & Shaver, 1994). This kind of caregiving may be exhausting for both parties. We have demonstrated in patient–caregiver dyads that caregivers with less attachment security are more likely to become depressed, even after controlling for the objective and subjective burdens of caregiving (Braun et al., 2007, 2012).

Attachment theory can help healthcare providers understand and respond more effectively to the distress and behavior of dying patients and families seen in clinics, in palliative care, or in intensive care units (Curtis et al., 2012; Petersen & Koehler, 2006). The framework highlights that patients and families benefit from the secure base provided by relationships with healthcare providers who are attuned and responsive to their unique needs, recognizing that these may change with growing threats and new challenges. Attachment theory may also draw attention to the different relational needs of those who tend to be avoidantly or anxiously attached and those with paradoxically high levels of both attachment avoidance and anxiety (Tan et al., 2005).

ATTACHMENT AND CALM

Psychotherapeutic interventions such as CALM, which are focused on the restoration and maintenance of attachment security, may have particular value in the context of advanced disease. The attachment style of the patient may first become evident in the nature of the relationship established with the therapist. Some individuals are cautious about allowing an emotional connection, while others are more readily able to accept and receive support. These differences may also be apparent in the patient's family relationships, in which there may be greater or lesser degrees of intimacy and autonomy. Although patients can and often do experience equilibrium in and satisfaction with several important attachment relationships, these may be disrupted in the context of advanced cancer. Due to the increasing dependency and emotional distress associated with advanced disease, patients may require more emotional support from partners, family members, or friends. Renegotiation of important attachment relationships in this circumstance may require patients to accept and articulate their needs more clearly. Partners and family members may also need to adapt to the patient's needs more flexibly. CALM can help in this renegotiation, which may include sessions with the patient and their partner, family member, or friend. Discussion about sensitive issues in therapy may also support patients in communicating their feelings more easily to their loved ones.

The shifts in attachment relationships that may occur over the course of CALM therapy can sometimes be profound and dramatic. We have seen partners who were more removed and autonomous become more intimately engaged with their loved one in the context of advanced disease. This may be due to a heightened awareness of the needs of their partner, which may be furthered as a result of the patient identifying and communicating their needs with more clarity.

However, it is important to note that these shifts do not always occur, and there may be great sadness and feelings of isolation on the part of patients when their attachment relationships do not change as desired. In these cases, other family members, friends, or the therapist may become the most important source(s) of attachment security for the patient. Attachment security in the therapeutic relationship is essential for patients to reflect on their experiences and consider multiple perspectives, a process which is captured in the construct of mentalization (see Chapter 5 of this volume). The clinical application of attachment security and mentalization are described in more depth in Part II of this book.

CONCLUSION

Attachment security is fundamental to the relief of distress and to the maintenance of psychological well-being. Advanced disease activates the attachment system, and those who are less securely attached are more likely to experience distress and to have difficulty in renegotiating their attachment relationships at this time of heightened need. The relationship between patients and therapists may provide attachment security for those facing advanced disease and may also assist in the renegotiation of other important attachment relationships. This is often a critically important task for individuals facing advanced illness because of the increased dependency, loss of autonomy, and heightened requirements for emotional support in both patients and caregivers in this context. An attachment-based therapy such as CALM supports mentalization and draws attention to this important dimension in the psychosocial care of individuals with advanced disease.

REFERENCES

Bowlby, J. (1969). *Attachment and loss*. Vol. 1: *Attachment*. Hogarth Press and the Institute of Psycho-Analysis.

Bowlby, J. (1973). *Attachment and loss*. Vol. 2: *Separation, anxiety and anger*. Hogarth Press and the Institute of Psycho-Analysis.

Bowlby, J. (1980). *Attachment and loss*. Vol. 3: *Loss: Sadness and depression*. Hogarth Press and Institute of Psycho-Analysis.

Braun, M., Hales, S., Gilad, L., Mikulincer, M., Rydall, A., & Rodin, G. (2012). Caregiving styles and attachment orientations in couples facing advanced cancer. *Psycho-Oncology, 21*(9), 935–943.

Braun, M., Mikulincer, M., Rydall, A., Walsh, A., & Rodin, G. (2007). Hidden morbidity in cancer: Spouse caregivers. *Journal of Clinical Oncology, 25*(30), 4829–4834.

Brennan, K. A., Clark, C. L., & Shaver, P. R. (1998). Self-report measurement of adult romantic attachment: An integrative overview. In J. A. Simpson & W. S. Rholes (Eds.), *Attachment theory and close relationships* (pp. 46–76). The Guilford Press.

Burke, B. L., Martens, A., & Faucher, E. H. (2010). Two decades of terror management theory: A meta-analysis of mortality salience research. *Personality and Social Psychology Review, 14*(2), 155–195.

Chochinov, H. M., Hack, T., McClement, S., Kristjanson, L., & Harlos, M. (2002). Dignity in the terminally ill: A developing empirical model. *Social Science & Medicine, 54*(3), 433–443.

Curtis, J. R., Ciechanowski, P. S., Downey, L., Gold, J., Nielsen, E. L., Shannon, S. E., Treece, P. D., Young, J. P., & Engelberg, R. A. (2012). Development and evaluation of an interprofessional communication intervention to improve family outcomes in the ICU. *Contemporary Clinical Trials, 33*(6), 1245–1254.

Evans, A. J. (1994). Anticipatory grief: A theoretical challenge. *Palliative Medicine, 8*(2), 159–165.

Fraley, R. C., Waller, N. G., & Brennan, K. A. (2000). An item-response theory analysis of self-report measures of adult attachment. *Journal of Personality and Social Psychology, 78*(2), 350–365.

Ganzini, L., Goy, E. R., & Dobscha, S. K. (2009). Oregonians' reasons for requesting physician aid in dying. *Archives of Internal Medicine, 169*(5), 489–492.[Erratum in: *Archives of Internal Medicine,* 2009 Mar 23, 169(6), 57].

George, C., Kaplan, N., & Main, M. (1996). *Adult attachment interview* [Unpublished manuscript]. Department of Psychology, University of California.

Glajchen, M. (2004). The emerging role and needs of family caregivers in cancer care. *The Journal of Supportive Oncology, 2*(2), 145–155.

Greenberg, J. (2012). Terror management theory: From genesis to revelations. In P. R. Shaver & M. Mikulincer (Eds.), *Meaning, mortality, and choice: The social psychology of existential concerns* (pp. 17–35). American Psychological Association.

Grunfeld, E., Coyle, D., Whelan, T., Clinch, J., Reyno, L., Earle, C. C., Willan, A., Viola, R., Coristine, M., Janz, T., & Glossop, R. (2004). Family caregiver burden: Results of a longitudinal study of breast cancer patients and their principal caregivers. *CMAJ: Canadian Medical Association Journal, 170*(12), 1795–1801.

Hunter, M. J., Davis, P. J., & Tunstall, J. R. (2006). The influence of attachment and emotional support in end-stage cancer. *Psycho-Oncology, 15*(5), 431–444.

Johansson, Å. K., & Grimby, A. (2012). Anticipatory grief among close relatives of patients in hospice and palliative wards. *American Journal of Hospice and Palliative Medicine, 29*(2), 134–138.

Khan, L., Wong, R., Li, M., Zimmermann, C., Lo, C., Gagliese, L., & Rodin, G. (2010). Maintaining the will to live of patients with advanced cancer. *Cancer Journal, 16*(5), 524–531.

Kunce, L. J., & Shaver, P. R. (1994). An attachment-theoretical approach to caregiving in romantic relationships. In K. Bartholomew & D. Perlman (Eds.), *Advances in personal relationships, Vol. 5. Attachment processes in adulthood* (pp. 205–237). Jessica Kingsley Publishers.

Lo, C., Walsh, A., Mikulincer, M., Gagliese, L., Zimmermann, C., & Rodin, G. (2009). Measuring attachment security in patients with advanced cancer: Psychometric properties of a modified and brief Experiences in Close Relationships scale. *Psycho-Oncology, 18*(5), 490–499.

Main, M. (1995). Recent studies in attachment: Overview, with selected implications for clinical work. In S. Goldberg, R. Muir, & J. Kerr (Eds.), *Attachment theory: Social, developmental and clinical perspectives* (pp. 407–474). Analytics Press, Inc.

Maunder, R. G., & Hunter, J. J. (2016). Can patients be 'attached' to healthcare providers? An observational study to measure attachment phenomena in patient–provider relationships. *BMJ Open, 6*(5), e011068. doi: 10.1136/bmjopen-2016-011068.

McConnell, M., & Moss, E. (2011). Attachment across the life span: Factors that contribute to stability and change. *Australian Journal of Educational & Developmental Psychology, 11,* 60–77.

Parkes, C. M. (1996). Bereavement. *Studies in grief in adult life.* 3rd edition. Routledge.

Petersen, Y., & Koehler, L. (2006). Application of attachment theory for psychological support in palliative medicine during the terminal phase. *Gerontology, 52*(2), 111–123.

Rodin, G., Walsh, A., Zimmermann, C., Gagliese, L., Jones, J., Shepherd, F. A., Moore, M., Braun, M., Donner, A., & Mikulincer, M. (2007). The contribution of attachment security and social support to depressive symptoms in patients with metastatic cancer. *Psycho-Oncology, 16*(12), 1080–1091.

Tan, A., Zimmermann, C., & Rodin, G. (2005). Interpersonal processes in palliative care: An attachment perspective on the patient-clinician relationship. *Palliative Medicine, 19*(2), 143–150.

CHAPTER 5

Mentalization and Mortality

INTRODUCTION

Remaining engaged in life is no small feat for individuals with advanced cancer. Their lives are often dominated by physical limitations, clinic appointments, investigations and interventions, and dread that their next scan or test results will bring foreboding news. The all-encompassing world of cancer may collapse their identities and their relationships and may cause them to lose the imaginative capacity to readjust and reconfigure their lives. We have referred to the capacity to face advanced disease and the end of life while also attempting to live in a satisfying and meaningful way as "double awareness" (Rodin & Zimmermann, 2008). Without this capacity, individuals with advanced disease are at risk of relinquishing the life they could live, even when they are physically well enough to do so. The capacity to consider multiple perspectives is central to the concept of mentalization (Bateman & Fonagy, 2008). The focus in Managing Cancer and Living Meaningfully (CALM) on mentalization is intended to foster double awareness by helping patients to expand their view of themselves and of the possibilities that remain in their lives. In this chapter, we will elaborate on the concept of mentalization and its application to CALM therapy.

MENTALIZATION

The concept of mentalization emerged in the psychoanalytic literature in the 1960s, referring to a person's capacity to symbolize and to represent meaning (Freeman, 2016). It was subsequently refined to refer to the ability to reflect on and describe one's own mental states and those of others and to connect feelings, thoughts, and beliefs to behaviors (Bateman & Fonagy, 2008). Considering the multiple perspectives of another person and of oneself is an imaginative activity that requires more than direct observation (Bateman & Fonagy, 2008). Mentalization can be implicit, such as when we automatically and reflexively monitor and interpret what is in our mind, the mind of another, and the interplay between them (Davidsen & Fosgerau, 2015). It can also operate explicitly, when mental states and perspective-taking become the topic of conversation (Bateman & Fonagy, 2008).

The ability to mentalize develops in early childhood within the context of a secure attachment relationship (Bateman & Fonagy, 2013). It is facilitated by parental figures who attend to and mirror the feelings and experiences of the child. The primary failure of this capacity to develop is evident in conditions such as borderline personality disorder (Bateman & Fonagy, 2003). Individuals with this disorder tend to have difficulty differentiating between internal and external realities or experiencing or accepting any perspective other than their own (Bateman & Fonagy, 2008).

The capacity to mentalize varies on a continuum and may fluctuate according to the relational context, the affective state of the individual (Bateman & Fonagy, 2013), and the quality and nature of specific conversations (see Sperry, 2013). Although mentalization is often considered to be an individual capacity or characteristic, we have argued that it is also a relational construct that is co-produced within therapeutic conversations (Shaw et al., 2019; Shaw et al., 2020). To that end, we have conducted microscopic analyses of the conversations that have occurred within CALM to illuminate how therapists invite mentalization and how patients respond to and engage in mentalization talk. In the following paragraphs, we will explore mentalization in the context of therapeutic relationships, including those fostered in CALM, paying particular attention to the challenges that are unique to cancer.

MENTALIZATION IN THERAPY

Mentalization-based treatment was developed to help patients think about the way they and others think (Bateman & Fonagy, 2006). It has been successfully applied to a range of disorders, including depression (Bressi et al., 2017; Luyton et al., 2012), eating disorders (Robinson et al., 2016; Skårderud & Fonagy, 2012), and posttraumatic stress disorder (Allen et al.,

2012; Palgi et al., 2014). Since the consideration of multiple perspectives is most possible within a secure attachment relationship (Bateman & Fonagy, 2013), mentalization-based therapies involve providing a "secure base" for the patient. The therapist is curious, adopts a not-knowing stance about the patient's perspective, and works to avoid presuppositions or assumptions based on their own point of view or the objective reality of the situation. However, the therapist can sometimes articulate their own experience to present the possibility of an alternative mental state that is distinct from that of the patient and is not necessarily a direct representation of reality (Bateman & Fonagy, 2008). This may help to convey that there can be multiple perspectives on the same situation or circumstance.

MENTALIZATION IN ADVANCED CANCER

Mentalization in the context of advanced disease may pose unique challenges for both the patient and the therapist. Mortality may be difficult to mentalize because the distress generated by thoughts of death may interfere with the ability to think imaginatively and flexibly. Moreover, individuals may withhold their reflections on dying and death in therapeutic settings or in family relationships due to worries that their fears cannot be tolerated or managed by others. This may be particularly likely to occur when family or friends are unavailable or too overwhelmed themselves to provide assistance and support. One participant enrolled in CALM noted that when she mentioned her fears of dying to others: "It's a conversation stopper. You can't go any further."

Positive thinking has value in many circumstances, but it tends to fail in the context of advanced and progressive disease. One CALM participant said that when people tell her to "stay positive," it feels like "there's another expectation" put on her. The symptoms of the disease and living in the world of cancer can make it difficult for purely positive thinking to be sustained. The progression of disease and the proximity to the end of life also tend to narrow the possibilities for living, and alternative ways of living and thinking about the future may easily be obscured from both the patient and therapist (Hales & Rodin, 2021). Psychotherapeutic interventions in this context can help patients tolerate and manage their distress about dying and death and to consider the possibilities for living. This duality of managing the disease while engaging in life has previously been described in the thanatology and palliative care literature as "middle knowledge" (Weisman, 1972), as the "living–dying interval" (Pattison, 1977), and, more recently by our group, as "double awareness" (Rodin & Zimmermann,

2008). The CALM therapist does not aim to "correct" fears about mortality, but rather to expand awareness so that multiple perspectives on the present and the end of life can be entertained.

MENTALIZATION IN CALM THERAPY

CALM therapy helps to expand awareness by inviting reflection about all aspects of the patient's life and about the challenges of the disease and its progression. We have used the method of conversation analysis to elucidate the process through which therapists invite such reflection in CALM therapy. This methodology is uniquely designed to explore mentalization as a relational construct, through the moment-by-moment analysis of the connection in conversation between one utterance and the next (Shaw et al., 2020). Although we respond intuitively to one another in the moment, conversation analysis is a valuable tool to elucidate the details and nuances of interaction. The analysis relies on a transcription method that captures when talk is produced (e.g., after a pause or an overlap), the exact words used, and the intonation used to produce them (Jefferson, 2004). Dysfluencies and self-corrections in the interaction are important to capture as they show the speaker's self-awareness and attempt to make their talk understandable and acceptable to their recipient at the moment speech is produced (McCabe et al., 2016). The extracts presented here are simplified, illustrative transcripts, but some details, including the exact words used and overlapping talk, are included to illustrate relevant nuances within the conversations.

Whereas meaning is the primary *topic* for exploration in meaning-centered psychotherapy (see Breitbart, 2016), the exploration of meaning arises as a *process* between the therapist and patient in CALM, as in other so-called mentalization-based therapies. Engaging patients in the process of mentalization in CALM means supporting the consideration of alternative perspectives without dismissing the perspective presented by the patient. These additional perspectives are generally arrived at gradually through questions that first implicitly propose a different perspective but avoid the claim of superior knowledge (see Shaw et al., 2019). The patient's expressed perspective is accepted and validated, while other perspectives are also considered. In the following excerpt, the CALM therapist gradually guides the patient, who is reporting frustration with her partner, to a new perspective without invalidating the patient's original position.

Relationship Trouble

1 Th: So how does that cause a problem between the two of you?

2 P: Well it does with this illness, this is such an unpredictable course and you know, he likes to

3 plan his, he likes to travel he likes to plan his um, travel a year ahead and this is just one

4 example. Just he's a real planner and organizer and he's very social, he's been divorced for

5 many years and he developed a large network with friends and he likes to be around people

6 and um, he likes to just do a lot, and plan a lot and, I was okay with the, you know for the

7 most part, as long as we had um like time for ourselves, which we did, but since I've gotten sick I

8 don't feel like being around a lot of people all the time.

9 Th: How does he react to that?

10 P: Well he gets mad at me, he gets angry. We just had this two nights ago, this whole thing, I

11 mean I have good days and bad days, I have good weeks and bad weeks, when I go away

12 somewhere I'm able to like put it behind me for the most part and enjoy myself, but I– I'm not

13 the- same as I was three years ago.

14 Th: Do you believe he understands your condition?

15 P: Mm I don't—not fully. I don't think he understands it fully.

16 Th: A[ctually may]be I should ask you

17 P: [　Aha　]

18 P: [Do I] understand [it fully?　]

19 Th: [Wh–]　　　　　　[Or what] do you understand about it?

20 P: Well I know I have stage four lung cancer, but I'm, I feel good. I've gotta tell you. I'm not sick,

21 I've never been sick a day with this other than, psychological stuff, urm an' I I jus– I'm—tryna

22 fight it. An' I know that the stats are terrible, but I'm tryin' ta tell myself, unless it's zero

23 percent or a hundred percent, they don't count. An

24 Th: You're hoping you might beat this? Is that what you mean?

25 P: Or at least prolong my life, significantly with treatment. I don't think it's ever gonna be cured I—

26 I realize that, an' I'm told that at almost every session, I— or every appointment I have with

27   {Doctor Name}

28 Th: mm

29 P: She— says she can't cure me. But I urm, to the best of my knowledge I've 'ad a pretty good

30   response to the medication. I've never had a symptom, other than side effects of the

31   medication. Which I . . .

32 Th: Do you think that because you look, ur so normal, I don't know, feel normal, that—

33   [that—]

34 P: [I can't believe I'm so sick on paper and that I have a medical file that says that.

35 Th: And do you think that's why your husband has a hard time understanding it?

36 P: I don't know, maybe, I don't know, I've never thought of it.

The therapist responds to the patient's complaint about her husband with an enquiry about his understanding of her condition (line 14) and then about her own understanding (lines 16 & 19). These enquiries implicitly invite the patient to consider an alternative explanation for her husband's problematic behavior; specifically, she may not have conveyed the seriousness of her condition to her husband in a way that he fully understood or appreciated. The patient goes on to express that she knows that she has Stage IV lung cancer and that "the stats are terrible" (line 22) but that she is optimistic because she feels good (line 20). Once the patient has expanded on this perspective, the therapist more explicitly proposes that the husband's lack of understanding might actually be related to the patient's communication to him about her disease (lines 35).

It is noteworthy that the therapist explores an alternative perspective with the patient in a gradual way, first implicitly proposing that the patient's communications may have shaped the husband's limited understanding by merely enquiring into how they each understood her condition. Once the patient concedes that that her diagnosis actually seems incongruous to her, there is interactional space for the therapist to propose more explicitly that the husband's lack of understanding might be partly related to what the patient has communicated to him and how she appears. By arriving gradually at this perspective with the patient, the therapist is able to expand the patient's perspective without imposing on her a different point of view (see Shaw et al., 2019). The goal of the therapist is not to take sides in the conflict but to expand the range of options that can be considered to resolve the dilemma. It is possible that the patient is protecting both herself and her husband by not fully disclosing the extent of her disease, illustrating the system of mutual influence between patients and their partners (Lo et al., 2013).

A person's ability to mentalize at any moment in time is at least partly related to their relational context (Bateman & Fonagy, 2013) and to the quality and nature of the conversation in which they are engaged (Sperry, 2013). The therapist's own ability to mentalize therefore plays a role in the emergent mentalization capacity of the patient in CALM therapy, as it does in other mentalization-based therapies (Bateman & Fonagy, 2006). However, remaining open to multiple perspectives on living with advanced disease may be challenging for CALM therapists because of the shared knowledge about the disease and the threat of mortality. It may be difficult for patients and therapists to imagine alternative perspectives when the shadow of death looms so large. It may also be challenging to support the patient's engagement in life without seeming to dismiss their fears about dying and death.

In the following extract, another CALM participant describes difficulty remaining involved in family and work events when time seems so short.

Uncertainty and Loss

1 Th: There's a lot of uncertainty.
2 P: And a lot of potential loss.
3 Th: Yeah.
4 P: I don't think . . . I mean, I don't think that there's a whole lot of danger that I am gonna g– give up
5 and get depressed. I mean, it's kind of who I am. It is just getting my head around, a different
6 project I guess.
7 Th: Well you do feel sad. And it is sad.
8 P: Yes, I've been crying a lot.
9 Th: Yeah.
10 P: And so's {name} and so's {name} and so's {name}, we all feel sad. And we just have to get
11 through that. I– I mean it won't stay, I don't think. And then I felt anxious. Like, I couldn't
12 sleep last night. 'Cause all these questions I don't, you know, I don't have the answers to.
13 Th: I feel sad, an' there's uncertainty. Urm . . . there's always uncertainty but this,
14 P: (It should caught) up a [bit.]
15 Th: [Yah this,] ramps it up.

16 P: Y[eh.]

17 Th: [Yeah]

18 Th: Uhm I, an' about palliative care, I would see this as uh a– an insurance policy, uh

19   [that] they know you, an' that, if you should get symptoms, that– you'll get

20 P: [Yeah.]

21 Th: lots of help in managing them, [(now)]

22 P: [Yeah.]

23 Th: Uh . . . an' because that's wh– that—that helps, with the uncertainty, if [you know] what I

24 P: [Yeah]

25 Th: mean. To know that if you do have a symptom, that you won't be stuck with it.

26 P: Yeh.

27 Th: Uhm

28 P: (Yeh.)

29 Th: Uhm

30 P: Uhm I was trying to decide uh– I was thinking, that maybe it would be good if I took {name}

31   with me to that first appointment. But [(do they)]

32 Th: [I think] it's a good idea.

33 P: Is it ok?

34 Th: I think it's a good [idea]

35 P: [To do.]

36 P: 'Kay.

37 Th: They like that u– usually would prefer that.

The therapist validates the patient's experience, going so far as to label it as a fact: "It is sad." The patient then expands on these feelings, reporting that "we just have to get through that" (lines 10 and 11) but that she also feels anxious. The therapist again stays with these feelings, validating them and reporting them as if they were his own: "I feel sad and there's uncertainty" (line 13). However, the therapist goes on to propose that the palliative care services, which they had previously been talking about, could help with feelings of uncertainty about managing the symptoms (lines 18–25). Again, this is offered as an additional perspective, without objecting to the feeling of sadness and uncertainty expressed by the patient. By reintroducing palliative care, the therapist allows the patient to experience some sense of safety and security despite the uncertainty and progression of her disease. Holding this duality may be considered to reflect "double awareness."

The example here highlights the challenge that CALM therapists face in the task of validating feelings of sadness and hopelessness while also mentalizing alternative perspectives. Considering this extract in relation to the previous one highlights some of the complexity for the therapist of maintaining their own capacity to mentalize while also supporting that of the patient and their spouse.

MENTALIZATION AND THE RECLAIMING OF IDENTITY

One of the common complications of advanced cancer is the loss of identity, which may become collapsed and organized entirely around the disease. The next CALM therapy extract provides another example of how alternative perspectives can add to, rather than object to, the perspective of the patient. The patient describes the threat she experiences to her identity as a result of her condition. She expresses concern that she is being thought of primarily in terms of cancer and that she wants to "regain who she was" (line 12).

Cancer and Identity

1 P: Yeah. An' I think it's, it's a part of what felt endangered.
2 Th: Yes.
3 P: I– and, an' hard to get back.
4 Th: Yeah.
5 P: Mm
6 Th: Yeah.
7 P: Cos it feels like uh I thought, it is it's like so many of my colleagues have been so concerned an'
8   empathetic and,
9 Th: mm
10 P: And involved but I kina' like I wan' 'em t– not think of me as c[ancer.] I wan' ['em to]
11 Th: [Right.]   [Right.]
12 P: I wanna regain [who I] was.
13 Th: [Right.]
14 Th: Right.
15 P: But I don't know if I can do that.
16 P: It jus– you know, just like I don't know if I can take my life back. I don't know if I could

17   take myself back.
18 Th: You know– I would say the answer is somewhere in the middle, in the sense that if
19   you're going through all of this, it's hard to take cancer out of the equation all together.
20   Uhm our goal though is not— our goal maybe isn't to eliminate it all together, that you'll
21   never think about cancer, that's not possible, but that all of your thinking will be about
22   cancer, an' that some of what you hold on to is you. So okay you've got this disease, but
23   uhm that you can hold on to you, that is our [goal.] [An' it is a challenge.]
24 P: [Yeah.] [It's like—] [it's] like what uh well maybe a better
25   way of describing it is I need- I need to see- grow that space.
26   [(laugh)]
27 Th: [Yes] that's a very good [way of—] that's the [idea.]
28 P: [Yeah]   [Is– I—] I'm not gonna,
29 Th: Yeah.
30 P: get [it all] back, [but I] [need to grow] that [space.]
31 Th: [Right.]   [Yeah.]   [That's– that's a—
        [That's a beaut]iful way of putting it.
32 Th: That is exactly the goal.

The therapist responds to the patient by introducing a new way of thinking: that the patient can hold two representations of herself in mind at the same time (lines 18–23). The therapist accepts the patient's wish to "regain" herself and introduces the inevitability that some of her identity will continue to be linked to cancer. The patient then expands on this new way of thinking by describing the process as one of growth, rather than of fully regaining her former identity. This metaphor of "growing a space" captures the therapeutic process of mentalization in CALM of opening up imaginative possibilities for thinking.

SHIFTING FROM A FACT TO A FEELING

Exploring alternative perspectives with patients implicitly means distinguishing between feeling and fact. In the therapeutic situation, this involves enquiring about the implicit meaning of an utterance so that it is not treated as obvious and inevitable, but as one possible way of thinking about things (see Shaw et al., 2019). Identifying a perspective as a subjective feeling rather than a fact creates space for multiple and co-existing perspectives. The following extract provides an example of how a therapist implicitly and then explicitly invites consideration of a perspective as a feeling rather than a fact. The patient has received troubling news and articulates her perspective that she feels that she now must "give in" to her cancer, and let it take its course given the limited treatment options that are now available to her. We join the extract when the therapist seeks clarification from the patient regarding what counts as "giving in."

The meaning of "giving in"

1 Th: So having chemotherapy, means not giving in and not having chemotherapy means you're

2   giving in?

3 P: Uh yeah. I make a distinction between clinical trials an' chemo' yeah. But that's probably

4   splitting hairs. Yeah, it is how it feels. But—(well) . . . yeh. But then, I can't. I have to come to

5   terms with, an' accept that I'm gonna die—that I'm dying. Yeah. That's what it feels like I—

6   does it—it doesn't make sense to you? (laughter)

7 Th: Well it does an' it doesn't. I– I understand that it would feel better obviously, you'd feel

8   better an' be more encouraged, if the treatment was having an effect. Or better effect. I– I

9   understand that, but urm you know whether a drug is a good idea or whether it helps, is

10   sort of an empirical thing, I– I think when you talk about giving in ur that's a psychological

11   thing. An' I think the challenge now is to shift the idea of a project. A, part of me as I say,

12   [Doctor's name] will, an' will advise about the chemotherapy but I– I think it means sh– shifting

13   the project to you. An' helping you be as well as you can, whether or not you're receiving

14   chemotherapy.

15   (pause)

16 P: Yeh.

17 P: Yeah.

18 P: It makes sense. I'm so glad I have an appointment next Thursday, with the palliative care team.

19 Th: Oh good.

20 P: An' I'm glad that's in my book.

21 Th: Yeah.

22 P: 'Cause part of what I don't know is what that looks like. You know what that'll mean what it'll

23 translate in to in terms of things I c– can do, you know, uh an' I'm hoping that they'll also help

24 me with that.

The patient has recently received troubling news and has reported her feeling that she now must "give in" and let the cancer take its course, given her limited treatment options. By enquiring into the patient's meaning of "giving in" (lines 1-2), the therapist is treating the patient's perspective as not obvious or inevitable and therefore is implicitly proposing the possibility that there can be more than one way of considering things. We have proposed that these kinds of meaning expansion enquiries work to provide the patient with an opportunity to elaborate on their assumptions, allowing for an exploration of alternative perspectives (Shaw et al., 2019). As such, they implicitly shift the perspective from fact to feeling. It was only when the patient challenged the therapist (line 6) that the therapist more explicitly presented a different perspective, thereby explicitly separating fact from feeling; "giving in" is no longer treated as a necessary consequence of not receiving treatment. The therapist's talk is effective in enabling the patient to separate her feelings from fact. She reports that "it makes sense" (line 18) and goes on to report how she is glad to have an appointment with the palliative care team as they can help her identify the things she can do (lines 14–23). In other words, she is now considering a different project rather than just "giving in."

CONCLUSION

Patients with serious illnesses are often advised to think positively and maintain hope but, as they become more symptomatic, these strategies become unsustainable. Mentalization can help patients expand their view of the possibilities for living while facing the end of life. The CALM therapist aims to support this process without presuming what patients should experience. CALM clinicians aim to understand and empathize with death-related distress while also supporting experiences of resilience and strength in the face of this adversity. By fostering a consideration of multiple perspectives and shifting the patient's understanding of their viewpoint from a fact to a feeling, CALM facilitates discussions of fears, hopes, and possibilities and diminishes the terror and isolation of silence.

REFERENCES

Allen, J., Lemma, A., & Fonagy, P. (2012). Trauma. In A. Bateman & P. Fonagy (Eds.), *Handbook of mentalizing in mental health practice* (pp. 419–445). American Psychiatric Publishing, Inc.

Bateman, A. W., & Fonagy, P (2003). The development of an attachment-based treatment program for borderline personality disorder. *Bulletin of the Menninger Clinic, 67*(3), 187–211.

Bateman, A., & Fonagy, P. (2006). *Mentalization based treatment: A practical guide.* Oxford University Press.

Bateman, A., & Fonagy, P. (2008). Mentalization-based treatment for BPD. *Social Work in Mental Health, 6*(1–2), 187–201.

Bateman, A. W., & Fonagy, P. (2013). Mentalization-based treatment. *Psychoanalytic Inquiry, 33*(6), 595–613.

Breitbart, W. (Ed.). (2016). *Meaning-centered psychotherapy in the cancer setting: Finding meaning and hope in the face of suffering.* Oxford University Press.

Bressi, C., Fronza, S., Minacapelli, E., Nocito, E. P., Dipasquale, E., Magri, L., Lionetti, F., & Barone, L. (2017). Short-term psychodynamic psychotherapy with mentalization-based techniques in major depressive disorder patients: Relationship among alexithymia, reflective functioning, and outcome variables—A pilot study. *Psychology and Psychotherapy: Theory, Research and Practice, 90*(3), 299–313.

Davidsen, A. S., & Fosgerau, C. F. (2015). Grasping the process of implicit mentalization. *Theory & Psychology, 25*(4), 434–454.

Freeman, C. (2016). What is mentalizing? An overview. *British Journal of Psychotherapy, 32*(2), 189–201.

Hales, S., & Rodin, G. (2021). Managing Cancer And Living Meaningfully (CALM) therapy. In W. Breitbart, P. Butow, P. Jacobsen, W. Lam, M. Lazenby, & M. Loscalzo (Eds.). *Psycho-Oncology* Fourth edition. (pp. 487–491). Oxford University Press.

Jefferson, G. (2004). Glossary of transcript symbols with an introduction. In G. H. Lerner (Ed.), *Conversation analysis: Studies from the first generation* (pp. 13–31). John Benjamins Publishing Company.

Lo, C., Hales, S., Braun, M., Rydall, A. C., Zimmermann, C., & Rodin, G. (2013). Couples facing advanced cancer: Examination of an interdependent relational system. *Psycho-Oncology, 22*(10), 2283–2290.

Luyton, P., Fonagy, P., Lemma, A., & Target, M. (2012). Depression. In A. Bateman & P. Fonagy (Eds.), *Handbook of mentalizing in mental health practice* (pp. 385–418). American Psychiatric Publishing, Inc.

McCabe, R., John, P., Dooley, J., Healey, P., Cushing, A., Kingdon, D., Bremner, S., & Priebe, S. (2016). Training to enhance psychiatrist communication with patients with psychosis (TEMPO): Cluster randomised controlled trial. *The British Journal of Psychiatry, 209*(6), 517–524.

Palgi, S., Palgi, Y., Ben-Ezra, M., & Shrira, A. (2014). "I will fear no evil, for I am with me": Mentalization-oriented intervention with PTSD patients. A case study. *Journal of Contemporary Psychotherapy, 44*(3), 173–182.

Pattison, E. M. (1977). *The experience of dying.* Prentice Hall.

Robinson, P., Hellier, J., Barrett, B., Barzdaitiene, D., Bateman, A., Bogaardt, A., Clare, A., Somers, N., O'Callaghan, A., Goldsmith, K., Kern, N., Schmidt, U., Morando, S., Ouellet-Courtois, C., Roberts, A., Skårderud, F., & Fonagy, P. (2016). The NOURISHED randomised controlled trial comparing mentalisation-based treatment for eating disorders (MBT-ED) with specialist supportive clinical management (SSCM-ED) for patients with eating disorders and symptoms of borderline personality disorder. *Trials, 17*(1): 549. doi: 10.1186/s13063-016-1606-8.

Rodin, G., & Zimmermann, C. (2008). Psychoanalytic reflections on mortality: A reconsideration. *Journal of the American Academy of Psychoanalysis and Dynamic Psychiatry, 36*(1), 181–196.

Shaw, C., Chrysikou, V., Lanceley, A., Lo, C., Hales, S., & Rodin, G. (2019). Mentalization in CALM psychotherapy sessions: Helping patients engage with alternative perspectives at the end of life. *Patient Education and Counseling, 102*(2), 188–197.

Shaw, C., Lo, C., Lanceley, A., Hales, S., & Rodin, G. (2020). The assessment of mentalization: Measures for the patient, the therapist and the interaction. *Journal of Contemporary Psychotherapy, 50*(1), 57–65. https://doi.org/10.1007/s10879-019-09420-z

Skårderud, F., & Fonagy, P. (2012). Eating disorders. In A. Bateman & P. Fonagy (Eds.), *Handbook of mentalizing in mental health practice* (pp. 347–384). American Psychiatric Publishing, Inc.

Sperry, M. (2013). Putting our heads together: Mentalizing systems. *Psychoanalytic Dialogues, 23*(6), 683–699.

Weisman, A. D. (1972). *On dying and denying: A psychiatric study of terminality.* Behavioral Publications.

CHAPTER 6
Treatment Decisions and the Therapeutic Process

I don't think I really understood what committing to a trial really meant until I was part of that trial . . . It was far more than I was expecting.

—CALM participant

INTRODUCTION

Modern cancer care is intended to support the active participation of patients and families in decisions about the treatment that will be delivered. It aims to respect the autonomy of individuals who are receiving treatment, to encourage shared decision-making, and to ensure that informed consent is obtained. However, the goal of autonomy or even shared decision-making is somewhat illusory in a situation in which patients and families are distressed and desperate, and in which a meaningful understanding of the potential risks and benefits of an intervention are difficult to achieve. Further, brief appointments in busy cancer clinics often do not provide adequate time or space for patients to reflect on the risks and benefits of the treatment options presented to them and whether they are consistent with their own values and goals of care. This chapter outlines some of the unique aspects of treatment decision-making in the context of advanced cancer. It then describes how Managing Cancer and Living Meaningfully (CALM) may help patients to reflect in a neutral, unhurried space and consider the complex issues related to their treatment decisions.

The concept of informed consent in modern healthcare stresses the importance of the individual patient's ability to understand and appreciate information relevant to their illness and their treatment options. The medicolegal frameworks that surround this process typically emphasize the responsibility of healthcare providers to communicate information clearly and to allow patients to make decisions in line with their own personal beliefs and values. This process is intended to respect the autonomy of patients, a principle that is highly valued in many cultures and is particularly important in healthcare settings where decisions can have life and death implications.

The ethical principle of respect for autonomy is sometimes considered a requirement for informed consent to treatment or research to be legitimately obtained. From this perspective, autonomy means to recognize or decide for oneself what values, beliefs, commitments, and desires are important to guide action and decision-making. However, this perspective does not take into account the extent to which our thoughts and feelings are shaped by our relationships and social contexts. In some cultures, families become the unit of medical decision-making at some stages of disease (Chong et al., 2015), while in others, medical authority carries more weight (Ruhnke et al., 2000). Overall, the influence of family members, healthcare providers, and significant others on patients' decision-making is unavoidable, making the concept of autonomy much more ambiguous and highlighting the complexity of the process of informed consent.

Decision-making about treatment is further complicated when there is conflict about the best course of action. Healthcare providers, family members, and patients may differ in their opinion of the benefits of pursuing aggressive anticancer treatment or of the value of participating in phase I and phase II trials. Such differences are particularly likely to occur when there is ambiguity about the benefits and risks of the intervention, since most patients and families accept recommendations that are clear and unequivocal. Conflict in the decision-making process is considered external when it occurs among patients, family members, and healthcare providers (May, 2002; Carnevale, 2005). Internal conflict may also arise when individuals are themselves ambivalent about which course of action to pursue. Decision-making in the cancer treatment setting is difficult for patients when there is disagreement between themselves and their families or between themselves, their families, and their healthcare providers.

However, internal conflict may be equally challenging for patients who feel desperate about the course of their disease but are worried about the toxic effects of cancer treatment or uncertain whether the limited benefit that may result from a clinical trial is worth the risk and time commitment at this stage of their life. The profound emotional distress experienced by patients and their families and the potential shifts in their values and priorities as a result of the illness may create additional confusion and uncertainty about what decisions are most in line with these new values and beliefs.

A psychotherapeutic intervention such as CALM may help patients to address both internal and external conflict. The supportive aspects of the CALM relationship may assist with the regulation of intense affect and provide a reflective space in which patients may consider their own diverse feelings and disentangle them from the wishes and opinions of others. There is often not enough time in oncology clinics for such reflection to occur. Reflection of this kind involves considering the risks and benefits of further cancer treatment and finding ways of maintaining hope, whether further treatment is pursued or not. CALM sessions may also help patients clarify the questions that they want to ask their healthcare providers, which may be essential for their decision-making.

By supporting self-reflection and mentalization, CALM allows patients to think about and weigh their own wishes, fears, and preferences regarding treatment while also considering the perspectives of their family and healthcare providers. The goal is not for patients to make decisions that are independent of these other parties, but instead to better understand their own perspective and that of others in order to take the whole into account in their decisions. The relational support provided in CALM may help patients build a sense of competence and experience a greater sense of agency in their treatment decisions.

THERAPEUTIC MISCONCEPTION, MISESTIMATION, AND CLINICAL TRIALS

Decisions about treatment of metastatic cancer are most straightforward for patients when they have trusting relationships with their healthcare providers and have received clear evidenced-based recommendations. Decision-making is much more difficult when the likelihood of benefit from a treatment is ambiguous and when there may be considerable toxicity. In such cases, oncologists are also less likely to make clear recommendations and defer decision-making to patients.

Phase I and phase II trials represent the maximum point of uncertainty about the safety and utility of an intervention and about their risk–benefit ratio (Grankvist & Kimmelman, 2016). Although some patients may benefit from participating in such trials, the likelihood of benefit is small (Kimmelman, 2019). The primary aim of these trials is to determine toxicity and optimal dosage, and therefore the primary benefit is to future patients. Although some benefit may accrue to those participating in phase I and phase II trials, patients and families often have unrealistic expectations of their potential benefit or equate participation in these trials with maintaining hope and morale. They may misconstrue research as personal medical care, which has been termed "therapeutic misconception," or incorrectly estimate the chances of benefit and risk, termed "therapeutic misestimation." Both are common in patients with advanced cancer who enroll in phase I trials, even when there has been a thorough process of informed consent (Pentz et al., 2012). These factors make it difficult for patients to weigh the risks and benefits and to decide upon the treatment course that is best for them.

THE INFLUENCE OF DEATH-RELATED DISTRESS ON MEDICAL DECISION-MAKING

To what lengths patients should pursue anticancer treatment and phase I trials is one of the most difficult questions faced by patients, families, and healthcare providers. Such treatments may significantly prolong life and reduce symptoms but may also bring adverse effects due to their toxicity, particularly when they are delivered too close to the end of life. In fact, important indicators of the quality of care when approaching the end of life include less aggressive care (Bainbridge & Seow, 2016). "Aggressiveness of care" in this context refers to care that is of greater intensity, often with life-prolonging rather than palliative intent.

North American research suggests that care for patients with advanced cancer is becoming more aggressive (Ho et al., 2011), even though most patients who recognize that they are dying report wanting less aggressive care (Mack et al., 2010; Weeks et al., 1998). Less aggressive care is less costly (Cheung et al., 2015) and has been associated with better caregiver ratings of patient quality of life and quality of care, less caregiver bereavement-related distress (Prigerson et al., 2015; Wright et al., 2008, 2016; Zhang et al., 2012), and longer patient survival (Näppä et al.,

2011). Current guidelines recommend palliative care and advance care planning discussions early in the course of illness for patients with advanced cancer (Ferrell et al., 2017; Smith et al., 2012). This is based on strong evidence that early palliative care is associated with improved quality of life (Temel et al., 2010; Zimmermann et al., 2014), greater satisfaction with care (Zimmermann et al., 2014), less intensive oncological interventions, and prolonged survival (Temel et al., 2010). However, when palliative care referrals and advance care planning are delayed, more aggressive interventions are more likely to be delivered (Temel et al., 2010).

The factors that lead to the delivery of high-intensity medical care to patients with advanced cancer at the end of life require further elucidation. Patient and family attitudes and insistence on anticancer treatment to maintain hope and their readiness to face the end of life have been shown to influence communication and treatment choices (Innes & Payne, 2009). Similarly, healthcare provider, institutional, and/or healthcare system factors that support active intervention and avoidance of discussing the end of life may all play a role in encouraging more aggressive care (Dzeng et al., 2015).

Research on decision-making in the context of life-threatening illness has emphasized that distress about the end of life in patients, family members, and healthcare providers may influence treatment decisions and complicate the weighing of proposed options by patients. Both patients and clinicians may avoid advance care planning or discussion of palliative care referral, each waiting for the other party to address it. This mutual avoidance can become mutual collusion leading to more aggressive care, with less likelihood of referral to hospice or palliative care and less advance care planning (de Haes & Koedoot, 2003). In these situations, anticancer treatment may be used not only to treat the disease but also to provide hope and allay fears about the end of life. However, this approach may result in worse quality of life and poorer quality of dying and death. Addressing advance care planning and distress about dying and death in CALM can support decision-making and diminish the effects of fear and desperation on this process.

THE PROCESS OF PROGNOSTIC AWARENESS AND MORTALITY SALIENCE

The communication of prognostic information is a sensitive task for the clinicians delivering the news and for the patients receiving it (Chochinov et al., 2000; Glare et al., 2008). Research has shown that patients want to be informed about their prognosis, to the extent that this is possible, and that prognostic awareness is not inherently psychologically damaging (Barnett, 2006). In addition, the perspective that patients are either living or dying or either fighting cancer or giving up are false dichotomies that may lead to avoidance of advance care planning or referral to palliative care. Discussions about prognosis may be most effective when they are carried out in multiple conversations over time. Shifts in prognostic awareness typically occur when there is a transition in care or the onset of new physical symptoms. Viewing prognostic understanding as a process that develops over time may help patients, families, and healthcare providers to sustain "double awareness" (Rodin & Zimmermann, 2008), with a shifting view of what this means at different points in the disease trajectory.

THE BENEFIT OF A NEUTRAL SPACE FOR REFLECTION

Patients may benefit from time and a neutral space to reflect on the different ways to consider their situation and their treatment options. This opportunity may facilitate their understanding of their cancer and its treatment and help to clarify their personal beliefs and values. This is an important process, since the stakes are high for patients and their families when they decide to accept or decline aggressive anticancer treatment or participation in early-phase clinical trials. Reflective space provided by CALM within cancer treatment settings may be uniquely valuable in allowing them to consider these decisions from multiple perspectives. Patients value the CALM therapist's knowledge of the cancer care system, which allows them to understand the patient's experience more easily, without everything that patients are going through needing to be explained. Because CALM therapists are one step removed from cancer treatment decisions, they may be able to hold a more balanced stance, with less professional investment in a particular treatment course or path. The therapeutic process may then allow patients to consider both the risks and benefits of pursuing treatment, taking into account the views of their healthcare providers, families, and the online and public spaces to which many patients are exposed.

CONCLUSION

Decision-making about anticancer treatment is one of the most important tasks and challenges for patients with advanced disease. It is most straightforward when the indications for the treatment and the evidence of its beneficial effects are clear. However, when there is ambiguity about the likelihood of benefit of treatment, the values and preferences of patients and their families become even more important. This is particularly true in phase I trials, in which the likelihood of benefit is relatively small. CALM may be uniquely valuable in this setting because it provides the reflective space for patients to consider the risks and benefits of treatment options or clinical trials, which is not always available in oncology clinics. Engaging with patients in this process of decision-making, without imposing their own values or opinions, is one of the most challenging tasks for CALM therapists. Training in CALM and integration of therapists with both oncology and palliative care teams may help to maintain this delicate balance.

REFERENCES

Bainbridge, D., & Seow, H. (2016). Measuring the quality of palliative care at the end of life: An overview of data sources. *Healthy Aging & Clinical Care in the Elderly*, 8, 9–15.

Barnett, M. M. (2006). Does it hurt to know the worst? Psychological morbidity, information preferences and understanding of prognosis in patients with advanced cancer. *Psycho-Oncology*, 15(1), 44–55.

Carnevale, F. (2005). Ethical care of the critically ill child: A conception of a 'thick' bioethics. *Nursing Ethics*, 12(3), 239–252.

Cheung, M. C., Earle, C. C., Rangrej, J., Ho, T. H., Liu, N., Barbera, L., Saskin, R., Porter, J., Seung, S. J., & Mittmann, N. (2015). Impact of aggressive management and palliative care on cancer costs in the final month of life. *Cancer*, 121(18), 3307–3315.

Chochinov, H. M., Tataryn, D. J., Wilson, K. G., Enns, M., & Lander, S. (2000). Prognostic awareness and the terminally ill. *Psychosomatics*, 41(6), 500–504.

Chong, J. A., Quah, Y. L., Yang, G. M., Menon, S., & Krishna, L. K. R. (2015). Patient and family involvement in decision making for management of cancer patients at a centre in Singapore. *BMJ Supportive & Palliative Care*, 5(4), 420–426. http://dx.doi.org/10.1136/bmjspcare-2012-000323.

de Haes, H., & Koedoot, N. (2003). Patient centered decision making in palliative cancer treatment: A world of paradoxes. *Patient Education and Counseling*, 50(1), 43–49.

Dzeng, E., Smith, T. J., & Levine, D. M. (2015). What are the contributing factors towards overly aggressive care at the end of life? *Journal of General Internal Medicine*, 30, S301.

Ferrell, B. R., Temel, J. S., Temin, S., Alesi, E. R., Balboni, T. A., Basch, E. M., Firn, J. I., Paice, J. A., Peppercorn, J. M., Phillips, T., Stovall, E. L., Zimmermann, C., & Smith, T. J. (2017). Integration of palliative care into standard oncology care: American Society of Clinical Oncology Clinical Practice Guideline Update. *Journal of Clinical Oncology*, 35(1), 96–112.

Glare, P., Sinclair, C., Downing, M., Stone, P., Maltoni, M., & Vigano, A. (2008). Predicting survival in patients with advanced disease. *European Journal of Cancer*, 44(8), 1146–1156.

Grankvist, H., & Kimmelman, J. (2016). How do researchers decide early clinical trials? *Medicine, Health Care, and Philosophy, 19*(2), 191–198.

Ho, T. H., Barbera, L., Saskin, R., Lu, H., Neville, B. A., & Earle, C. C. (2011). Trends in the aggressiveness of end-of-life cancer care in the universal health care system of Ontario, Canada. *Journal of Clinical Oncology, 29*(12), 1587–1591.

Innes, S., & Payne, S. (2009). Advanced cancer patients' prognostic information preferences: A review. *Palliative Medicine, 23*(1), 29–39.

Kimmelman, J. (2019). Phase I trials as therapeutic options: (Usually) a betrayal of evidence-based medicine. *Nature Reviews Clinical Oncology, 16*(12), 719–720.

Mack, J. W., Weeks, J. C., Wright, A. A., Block, S. D., & Prigerson, H. G. (2010). End-of-life discussions, goal attainment, and distress at the end of life: Predictors and outcomes of receipt of care consistent with preferences. *Journal of Clinical Oncology, 28*(7), 1203–1208.

May, T. (2002). *Bioethics in a liberal society: The political framework of bioethics decision making*. Johns Hopkins University Press.

Näppä, U., Lindqvist, O., Rasmussen, B. H., & Axelsson, B. (2011). Palliative chemotherapy during the last month of life. *Annals of Oncology, 22*(11), 2375–2380.

Pentz, R. D., White, M., Harvey, R. D., Farmer, Z. L., Liu, Y., Lewis, C., Dashevskaya, O., Owonikoko, T., & Khuri, F. R. (2012). Therapeutic misconception, misestimation, and optimism in participants enrolled in phase 1 trials. *Cancer, 118*(18), 4571–4578.

Prigerson, H. G., Bao, Y., Shah, M. A., Paulk, M. E., LeBlanc, T. W., Schneider, B. J., Garrido, M. M., Reid, M. C., Berlin, D. A., Adelson, K. B., Neugut, A. I., & Maciejewski, P. K. (2015). Chemotherapy use, performance status, and quality of life at the end of life. *JAMA Oncology, 1*(6), 778–784.

Rodin, G., & Zimmermann, C. (2008). Psychoanalytic reflections on mortality: A reconsideration. *Journal of the American Academy of Psychoanalysis and Dynamic Psychiatry, 36*(1), 181–196.

Ruhnke, G. W., Wilson, S. R., Akamatsu, T., Kinoue, T., Takashima, Y., Goldstein, M. K., Koenig, B. A., Hornberger, J. C., & Raffin, T. A. (2000). Ethical decision making and patient autonomy: A comparison of physicians and patients in Japan and the United States. *Chest, 118*(4), 1172–1182.

Smith, T. J., Temin, S., Alesi, E. R., Abernethy, A. P., Balboni, T. A., Basch, E. M., Ferrell, B. R., Loscalzo, M., Meier, D. E., Paice, J. A., Peppercorn, J. M., Somerfield, M., Stovall, E., & Von Roenn, J. H. (2012). American Society of Clinical Oncology provisional clinical opinion: The integration of palliative care into standard oncology care. *Journal of Clinical Oncology, 30*(8), 880–887.

Temel, J. S., Greer, J. A., Muzikansky, A., Gallagher, E. R., Admane, S., Jackson, V. A., Dahlin, C.M., Blinderman, C.D., Jacobsen, J., Pirl, W.F., Billings, J. A., & Lynch, T. J. (2010). Early palliative care for patients with metastatic non–small-cell lung cancer. *The New England Journal of Medicine, 363*(8), 733–742.

Weeks, J. C., Cook, E. F., O'Day, S. J., Peterson, L. M., Wenger, N., Reding, D., Harrell, F. E., Kussin, P., Dawson, N. V., Connors Jr, A. F., Lynn, J. , & Phillips, R. S. (1998). Relationship between cancer patients' predictions of prognosis and their treatment preferences. *JAMA, 279*(21), 1709–1714.

Wright, A. A., Keating, N. L., Ayanian, J. Z., Chrischilles, E. A., Kahn, K. L., Ritchie, C. S., Weeks, J. C., Earle, C. C., & Landrum, M. B. (2016). Family perspectives on aggressive cancer care near the end of life. *JAMA, 315*(3), 284–292.

Wright, A. A., Zhang, B., Ray, A., Mack, J. W., Trice, E., Balboni, T., Mitchell, S.L.,
Jackson, V.A., Block, S.D., Maciejewski, P.K., & Prigerson, H. G. (2008).
Associations between end-of-life discussions, patient mental health, medical
care near death, and caregiver bereavement adjustment. *JAMA, 300*(14),
1665–1673.

Zhang, B., Nilsson, M. E., & Prigerson, H. G. (2012). Factors important to patients'
quality of life at the end of life. *Archives of Internal Medicine, 172*(15),
1133–1142.

Zimmermann, C., Swami, N., Krzyzanowska, M., Hannon, B., Leighl, N., Oza, A.,
Moore, M., Rydall, A., Rodin, G., Tannock, I., Donner, A., & Lo, C. (2014).
Early palliative care for patients with advanced cancer: A cluster-randomised
controlled trial. *The Lancet, 383*(9930), 1721–1730.

CHAPTER 7
CALM and the Desire for Death

I've experienced such incredible pain over the last little while and more in the last week. Such incredible pain that it made me think that death is preferable to this.
—Will to Live study participant

INTRODUCTION

Psychological disturbances in patients with advanced cancer may manifest not only as symptoms of distress but also as the loss of the will to live or as the desire for death (Khan et al., 2010). The will to live, which has been defined as the psychological expression of the striving for life, has rational, emotional, and instinctual underpinnings (Carmel, 2001). Although patients may question the value of life in the face of significant suffering or disability, the will to live is nevertheless preserved in most individuals with advanced disease (Rodin et al., 2007), even in palliative care settings (Chochinov et al., 1995). Since the loss of the will to live is not inevitable in advanced cancer, it deserves explanation and potential therapeutic intervention when it arises.

The loss of the will to live may present as apathy, resignation, welcoming the relief from suffering, or as implicit or explicit desires for death. It can be difficult to distinguish the loss of the will to live as a manifestation of depression from nonpathological death acceptance or "rational suicide" (Cheung et al., 2017). The difficulty in making this distinction in individuals with advanced disease has become even more relevant with the recent legalization of assisted dying in many jurisdictions. Such legislation reflects a dramatic shift in societal attitudes, laws, and policies related to the ability of patients to choose to end their lives (Chochinov et al., 1995; Johansen et al., 2005). However, these policies may not fully take into account the complexity of the motivation that leads individuals to make such decisions.

At this time, some form of assisted dying has been legalized in the Netherlands, Belgium, Colombia, Luxembourg, Switzerland, Germany, Canada, the State of Victoria in Australia, New Zealand, and in eight jurisdictions in the United States: Oregon (1994), Washington (2008), Montana (2009), Vermont (2013), California (2015), Colorado (2016), the District of Columbia (2016), and Hawaii (2018; Emanuel et al., 2016; Steck et al., 2013). Evidence from these regions indicates that many more patients with advanced disease consider physician-assisted death than ultimately follow through with it (Blanke et al., 2017; Tolle et al., 2004). Further, although rates of assisted death tend to increase in countries where it is legalized, it still accounts for only 0.1% to 4.6% of all deaths in these jurisdictions (Radbruch et al., 2016).

Medical assistance in dying, referred to by its acronym MAiD, became legal for adults in Canada in 2016. Key eligibility criteria in the original federal legislation included the capacity to provide informed consent, a reasonably foreseeable natural death, and physical or psychological suffering that is intolerable to the individual. Revisions to the Canadian legislation have since been proposed to remove from the eligibility criteria the need for a reasonably foreseeable natural death and to allow for advance directives for MAiD under certain circumstances, unless the patient appears to object or refuse the procedure at the moment of the intervention (Government of Canada, 2020). However, distinguishing "rational" requests for assisted dying from a psychological disturbance warranting intervention in the context of advanced cancer is no small task. This chapter will explore the desire for death in advanced cancer and the potential role of Managing Cancer and Living Meaningfully (CALM) therapy in addressing this state.

THE DESIRE FOR DEATH IN ADVANCED CANCER

In the Will to Live study (see Chapter 3 of this volume), a high desire for death was found in only 1.5% of patients with metastatic cancer (Rodin et al., 2007). The infrequency of the desire for death in such patients may not be surprising, since all had sought active treatment at a major comprehensive cancer center. However, symptoms of hopelessness, depression, and impaired functional status were more common among those who reported a high desire for hastened death than in the rest of the sample. In research conducted by others with patients with advanced cancer, many of whom were receiving home or inpatient palliative care, 12% reported a high desire for death (Wilson et al., 2016); these individuals also reported more severe symptoms of distress and greater functional impairment. These findings suggest that the rational desire to end life is uncommon, even with advanced disease and proximity to death but, when present, may be entangled with physical and psychological suffering.

The desire for death in individuals with advanced disease is perhaps the least ambiguous in those who act upon this desire by committing suicide. Recent studies have shown that the overall risk of suicide in individuals with cancer is up to four times that in the general population and much higher in those with advanced disease (Kaceniene et al., 2017; Misono et al., 2008; Saad et al., 2019; Zaorsky et al., 2019). Even more striking, Fang and colleagues (2012) found that in the first week following a diagnosis of advanced disease, the risks of suicide and of cardiac death are, respectively, 12 and 5 times higher than in the general population. These risks are again highest in those with more advanced disease (Misono et al., 2008). Requests for assistance in dying in countries where it has been legalized are made predominantly by individuals with advanced cancer (Blanke et al., 2017; Emanuel et al., 2016; Li et al., 2017; Steck et al., 2013). The reasons for the preponderance of cancer in assisted death are not well understood but could be due to the anticipated or actual symptom burden, the predictable disease course, the capacity to provide informed consent until near the end of life, and the greater access of patients with cancer to specialized palliative and end-of-life care, compared to those with other advanced diseases (Pardon et al., 2013).

There is evidence that the desire for death and the will to live fluctuate significantly over time (Chochinov et al., 1995; Hudson et al., 2006; Johansen et al., 2005; Rodin et al., 2007), even during the last few weeks of life (Rosenfeld et al., 2014). This was demonstrated in a study of almost 1,000 American patients with advanced disease in which more than 10% reported seriously considering euthanasia or physician-assisted dying (Rosenfeld et al., 2014). When reassessed two to six months later, approximately half of those who had been considering such interventions had changed their minds, and an almost equal number who had not endorsed them originally were then seriously considering them. This degree of fluctuation suggests that the will to live and the desire for death in individuals with advanced disease may be influenced by a variety of factors that include their psychological state, the adequacy of their symptom control, their functional capacity, and their social context. It may also mean that the desire for death may be ameliorated by a psychotherapeutic intervention such as CALM.

THE MEANING OF THE LOSS OF THE WILL TO LIVE AND
THE DESIRE FOR DEATH

The will to live refers to a motivational state within an individual but is closely linked to the individual's social context and to their sense of connection to others. This was noted in inpatient palliative care settings, where the will to live was most likely to be sustained in those who were socially embedded (Tataryn & Chochinov, 2002). Expectations of support, reflected in attachment security (see Chapter 4 of this volume), may be even more important than actual social support received in preserving the will to live. Those who lack attachment security may fear the imposed dependency of advanced disease and have less capacity to renegotiate relationships in this new circumstance. Although assisted dying is often framed as an intervention to relieve physical suffering or to preserve dignity in the context of advanced disease (Attaran, 2015), requests for assisted dying may equally reflect the wish to avoid the increasing dependency that occurs with progressive illness by prematurely ending life. In that regard, a relationship has been demonstrated between attachment avoidance and both the wish to hasten death and requests for assisted dying (Oldham et al., 2011; Rodin et al., 2009; Smith et al., 2015). Age and other sociodemographic factors may also affect the will to live and the desire for death (Carmel, 2001), with rational suicide being more common in older individuals (Cheung et al., 2017).

There have been concerns that the legalization of assisted dying would lead to the neglect of palliative care and that untreated suffering would cause more individuals with advanced disease to seek assisted dying (Barutta & Vollmann, 2015; Radbruch et al., 2016). These fears have thus far not materialized, in that the legalization of assisted dying has not diminished attention to palliative care (Chambaere & Bernheim, 2015). Some research has shown that patients who seek assisted dying have even greater access to palliative care than do other individuals with advanced disease (Dierickx et al., 2018). This suggests that assisted dying is more often sought for psychological reasons than to relieve current physical suffering.

Qualitative interviews conducted in the Will to Live study revealed that the desire for death in the context of advanced cancer is subsumed under three distinct, but not mutually exclusive, categories that fluctuate over time (Nissim et al., 2009). The most common and persistent experience of the desire for hastened death is as a hypothetical exit plan. This involves contemplating the hastening of death not as a present option, but as a future plan to be activated when all other means of controlling the illness have failed. From this perspective, hastening death is viewed as a reassurance that individuals could avoid an unwanted dying phase if they so wished. As one patient explained, "I have lots to live for, but if I come to the point when I'm too weak to do anything then I don't want to stay." Paradoxically, the sense of cognitive mastery that is derived from contemplating this hypothetical exit plan (a "Plan B") allows these individuals to maintain their commitment to continuing with life-prolonging treatment.

The desire for death was also considered by patients as a means of relieving overwhelming feelings of despair, hopelessness, and panic (Nissim et al., 2009). This feared state was described by one participant as being "in a dark tunnel, without seeing any light." Others described it as a "vicious cycle" and as a "paralysis from which the only way out is death." One patient said,

> Just let me die. I don't want to have to wake up and face this. I pray that I would just die in my sleep. I have nothing to live for, absolutely nothing. There's nothing coming up in my life that I'm living towards, and if there was it would be so terrible because it probably wouldn't happen.

Similar states of despair were described by many participants, although most were transient. Typically, the desire for hastened death in this circumstance was triggered by a stressful event, such as a disappointing test result, or an exacerbation of physical symptoms, particularly pain. The sense of despair in this context was often heightened by feelings of isolation and helplessness and sometimes triggered by the inability to access healthcare services or providers. Recovery from this state was often tied to a sense of familial connection, with some patients stating that the reason that they held onto life was because of the importance of their connection and commitment to their partner, children, and grandchildren. This recovery may be facilitated by invitations to mentalize or to consider alternate perspectives in a safe, reflective space (see Chapter 5 of this volume), sometimes liberating them from "the dark tunnel, without any light."

Finally, the desire for hastened death was sometimes experienced as a form of "letting go." This occurred most often in the active dying phase of the illness. One patient explained, "I realize that my time has come," and described this final stage as comforting and welcomed, reporting that many aspects of life that were previously considered important were now experienced as bothersome. Such individuals often reported feeling too tired to have visitors, and medical interventions began to seem pointless to them. As one patient said, "There are limits to what any organism will take or can do, and I have reached my limit." Another patient who was religious said, "We have to accept the fact that there is no miracle here—that my time is over." The death preparation that is facilitated by CALM therapy may help patients with advanced disease achieve this state of equanimity at the end of life.

Distinguishing between the three distinct experiences of the desire for hastened death—cognitive mastery or "Plan B," despair, or death acceptance—has important theoretical and clinical implications. The reflective space provided by CALM may allow elucidation of these states and relief from the distress associated with them. Indeed, the communication of these feelings to an empathic listener may be the most important therapeutic intervention in CALM and in conversations with medical providers. Novel approaches are now being developed to educate medical providers about how to engage in such conversations (Gewarges et al., 2020).

THE POTENTIAL ROLE OF CALM IN THE DESIRE FOR DEATH

There has been extensive research and clinical attention directed to the assessment of the competency of those who request assisted dying and whether they suffer from comorbid psychiatric disorders. However, there has been much less attention to the meaning of these requests and whether psychotherapeutic interventions can ameliorate the desire for death or loss of the will to live. CALM is designed to address these concerns and others that may lead to the loss of the will to live or the desire for death. The potential role of CALM in directly or indirectly addressing the desire for death as it relates to each of the four CALM domains is addressed here and summarized in Table 7.1.

CALM is intended to improve communication of patients with their healthcare providers so that there can be optimal control of their physical symptoms, shared decision-making, and goals of care consistent with their own values and wishes (see Chapter 6 of this volume). Attention to attachment security and to the renegotiation of attachment relationships as dependency needs grow—a central focus of CALM—may help to relieve dependency fears and to ensure optimal support from family members and healthcare providers (see Chapter 4 of this volume). Addressing issues related to the sense of meaning in their lives and to their fears, hopes, and wishes for the future may also diminish distress related to the end of life. For many patients, this is the first opportunity that they have had to discuss their will to live or desire for death and to consider assisted dying as one of their many possible options. One patient who considered MAiD to avoid the kind of death that he observed in his father was relieved to learn

Table 7.1. CALM DOMAINS AND THEIR POTENTIAL APPLICATION
FOR REDUCING THE DESIRE FOR DEATH

Domain	1. Symptom Management and Communication With Healthcare Providers	2. Changes in Self and Relations With Close Others	3. Spirituality and Sense of Meaning and Purpose	4. Preparing for the Future, Hope and Mortality
Focus of discussions in this domain	Cooperation and improvement of communication with healthcare providers, and help regarding medical decision-making to ensure best care and control of symptoms	Supporting the adjustment in self-esteem, identity, and relationships with close others that are required as a result of cancer-related changes	Reconsideration of life priorities and goals in the context of advanced disease	Acknowledgment of anticipatory fears, sustaining "double awareness," and planning for disease progression and the end of life
Aim of this domain	Attention to the practical problems and treatment decisions that individuals must face, and to their relationships with healthcare providers	Attention to adjustment disruptions in attachment security, and to the renegotiation of attachment relationships that is often required in advanced cancer	Reconsideration and reframing of life priorities	To face fears and make plans for the progression of disease and plan for the end of life
Potential application of each domain for the desire for death	Patients who feel empowered to address their healthcare providers are more likely to have their symptoms well-managed, to have treatment that is better aligned with their values, and to feel a greater sense of control	The restoration of self-esteem, the bolstering of attachment security, and the renegotiation of attachment relationships all may diminish death anxiety and the desire for death	The reframing of life priorities and the reflection on life as it has been lived until this moment may restore hope and morale and diminish the desire for death	The opportunity to communicate fears related to dying and death and to discuss planning for the end of life may help to diminish death anxiety and the desire for death

that a residential hospice might provide the kind of end-of-life care that he sought, without burdening his family.

It is possible that psychotherapeutic interventions such as CALM may alleviate the desire for death and enhance the will to live either directly or indirectly through its effect on the treatment and prevention of depression. However, this is not yet known, since almost half of individuals who request assisted dying in our cancer center do not accept or are not referred for specialized psychosocial care (Li et al., 2017). It is therefore not yet clear whether early implementation of CALM will diminish the desire for assisted death or requests for assisted dying in these individuals. We hope to clarify this in a large longitudinal study that we are conducting to identify more clearly the predictors of the desire for death and requests for medical assistance in dying and to determine the effect of CALM and other interventions on these outcomes.

CONCLUSION

The desire for death and the loss of the will to live may be secondary to physical or psychological suffering or to the fears of such outcomes, particularly in individuals who tend to be avoidantly attached. These states may be alleviated or modified by therapeutic interventions, in contrast to states of death acceptance associated with so-called rational suicide. CALM can provide individuals facing the end of life with the reflective space needed to consider the possibilities for the time that remains and to contemplate the meaning of the loss of the will to live and the desire for death if and when it emerges. Further prospective research is now underway to determine to what extent CALM can prevent or delay the loss of the will to live and the desire for death in patients with advanced disease.

REFERENCES

Attaran, A. (2015). Unanimity on death with dignity—Legalizing physician-assisted dying in Canada. *The New England Journal of Medicine, 372*(22), 2080–2082.

Barutta, J., & Vollmann, J. (2015). Physician-assisted death with limited access to palliative care. *Journal of Medical Ethics, 41*(8), 652–654.

Blanke, C., LeBlanc, M., Hershman, D., Ellis, L., & Meyskens, F. (2017). Characterizing 18 years of the Death with Dignity Act in Oregon. *JAMA Oncology, 3*(10), 1403–1406.

Carmel, S. (2001). The will to live: Gender differences among elderly persons. *Social Science & Medicine, 52*(6), 949–958.

Chambaere, K., & Bernheim, J. L. (2015). Does legal physician-assisted dying impede development of palliative care? The Belgian and Benelux experience. *Journal of Medical Ethics, 41*(8), 657–660.

Cheung, G., Douwes, G., & Sundram, F. (2017). Late-life suicide in terminal cancer: A rational act or underdiagnosed depression? *Journal of Pain and Symptom Management, 54*(6), 835–842.

Chochinov, H. M., Wilson, K. G., Enns, M., Mowchun, N., Lander, S., Levitt, M., & Clinch, J. J. (1995). Desire for death in the terminally ill. *The American Journal of Psychiatry, 152*(8), 1185–1191.

Dierickx, S., Deliens, L., Cohen, J., & Chambaere, K. (2018). Involvement of palliative care in euthanasia practice in a context of legalized euthanasia: A population-based mortality follow-back study. *Palliative Medicine, 32*(1), 114–122.

Emanuel, E. J., Onwuteaka-Philipsen, B. D., Urwin, J. W., & Cohen, J. (2016). Attitudes and practices of euthanasia and physician-assisted suicide in the United States, Canada, and Europe. *JAMA, 316*(1), 79–90.

Fang, F., Fall, K., Mittleman, M. A., Sparén, P., Ye, W., Adami, H. O., & Valdimarsdóttir, U. (2012). Suicide and cardiovascular death after a cancer diagnosis. *The New England Journal of Medicine, 366*(14), 1310–1318.

Gewarges, M., Gencher, J., Rodin, G., & Abdullah, N. (2020). Medical assistance in dying: A point of care educational framework for attending physicians. *Teaching and Learning in Medicine, 32*(2), 231–237.

Government of Canada. (2020, March 26). *Proposed changes to Canada's medical assistance in dying legislation*. Department of Justice. https://www.justice.gc.ca/eng/csj-sjc/pl/ad-am/index.html

Hudson, P. L., Kristjanson, L. J., Ashby, M., Kelly, B., Schofield, P., Hudson, R., Aranda, S., O'Connor, M., & Street, A. (2006). Desire for hastened death in patients with advanced disease and the evidence base of clinical guidelines: A systematic review. *Palliative Medicine, 20*(7), 693–701.

Johansen, S., Hølen, J. C., Kaasa, S., Loge, J. H., & Materstvedt, L. J. (2005). Attitudes towards, and wishes for, euthanasia in advanced cancer patients at a palliative medicine unit. *Palliative Medicine, 19*(6), 454–460.

Kaceniene, A., Krilaviciute, A., Kazlauskiene, J., Bulotiene, G., & Smailyte, G. (2017). Increasing suicide risk among cancer patients in Lithuania from 1993 to 2012: A cancer registry-based study. *European Journal of Cancer Prevention, 26*, S197–S203.

Khan, L., Wong, R., Li, M., Zimmermann, C., Lo, C., Gagliese, L., & Rodin, G. (2010). Maintaining the will to live of patients with advanced cancer. *Cancer Journal, 16*(5), 524–531.

Li, M., Watt, S., Escaf, M., Gardam, M., Heesters, A., O'Leary, G., & Rodin, G. (2017). Medical assistance in dying—Implementing a hospital-based program in Canada. *The New England Journal of Medicine, 376*(21), 2082–2088.

Misono, S., Weiss, N. S., Fann, J. R., Redman, M., & Yueh, B. (2008). Incidence of suicide in persons with cancer. *Journal of Clinical Oncology, 26*(29), 4731–4738.

Nissim, R., Gagliese, L., & Rodin, G. (2009). The desire for hastened death in individuals with advanced cancer: A longitudinal qualitative study. *Social Science & Medicine, 69*(2), 165–171.

Oldham, R. L., Dobscha, S. K., Goy, E. R., & Ganzini, L. (2011). Attachment styles of Oregonians who request physician-assisted death. *Palliative & Supportive Care, 9*(2), 123–128.

Pardon, K., Chambaere, K., Pasman, H. R. W., Deschepper, R., Rietjens, J., & Deliens, L. (2013). Trends in end-of-life decision making in patients with and without cancer. *Journal of Clinical Oncology, 31*(11), 1450–1457.

Radbruch, L., Leget, C., Bahr, P., Müller-Busch, C., Ellershaw, J., de Conno, F., Vanden Berghe, P., & Board Members of the EAPC. (2016). Euthanasia and physician-assisted suicide: A white paper from the European Association for Palliative Care. *Palliative Medicine, 30*(2), 104–116.

Rodin, G., Lo, C., Mikulincer, M., Donner, A., Gagliese, L., & Zimmermann, C. (2009). Pathways to distress: The multiple determinants of depression, hopelessness, and the desire for hastened death in metastatic cancer patients. *Social Science & Medicine, 68*(3), 562–569.

Rodin, G., Zimmermann, C., Rydall, A., Jones, J., Shepherd, F. A., Moore, M., Fruh, M., Donner, A., & Gagliese, L. (2007). The desire for hastened death in patients with metastatic cancer. *Journal of Pain and Symptom Management, 33*(6), 661–675.

Rosenfeld, B., Pessin, H., Marziliano, A., Jacobson, C., Sorger, B., Abbey, J., Olden, M., Brescia, R., & Breitbart, W. (2014). Does desire for hastened death change in terminally ill cancer patients? *Social Science & Medicine, 111*, 35–40.

Saad, A. M., Gad, M. M., Al-Husseini, M. J., AlKhayat, M. A., Rachid, A., Alfaar, A. S., & Hamoda, H. M. (2019). Suicidal death within a year of a cancer diagnosis: A population-based study. *Cancer, 125*(6), 972–979.

Smith, K. A., Harvath, T. A., Goy, E. R., & Ganzini, L. (2015). Predictors of pursuit of physician-assisted death. *Journal of Pain and Symptom Management, 49*(3), 555–561.

Steck, N., Egger, M., Maessen, M., Reisch, T., & Zwahlen, M. (2013). Euthanasia and assisted suicide in selected European countries and US states: Systematic literature review. *Medical Care, 51*(10), 938–944.

Tataryn, D., & Chochinov, H. M. (2002). Predicting the trajectory of will to live in terminally ill patients. *Psychosomatics, 43*(5), 370–377.

Tolle, S. W., Tilden, V. R., Drach, L. L., Fromme, E. K., Perrin, N. A., & Hedberg, K. (2004). Characteristics and proportion of dying Oregonians who personally consider physician-assisted suicide. *Journal of Clinical Ethics, 15*(2), 111–118.

Wilson, K. G., Dalgleish, T. L., Chochinov, H. M., Chary, S., Gagnon, P. R., Macmillan, K., De Luca, M., O'Shea, F., Kuhl, D., & Fainsinger, R. L. (2016). Mental disorders and the desire for death in patients receiving palliative care for cancer. *BMJ Supportive & Palliative Care, 6*(2), 170–177.

Zaorsky, N. G., Zhang, Y., Tuanquin, L., Bluethmann, S. M., Park, H. S., & Chinchilli, V. M. (2019). Suicide among cancer patients. *Nature Communications, 10*(1), 207. doi: 10.1038/s41467-018-08170-1.

CHAPTER 8

The Pearl in the Oyster

Posttraumatic Growth

I'm able to love you (my wife) deeper than before, I wish it didn't have to be this way.
—CALM participant

INTRODUCTION

The notion that trauma can promote psychological growth is widespread and offers an appealing silver lining for those who have suffered. This phenomenon, which has termed "posttraumatic growth" (PTG; Tedeschi & Calhoun, 2004) refers to the subjective experience of improved psychological well-being following highly distressing, traumatic experiences (Tedeschi & Calhoun, 2004; Zoellner & Maercker, 2006). PTG may manifest across five broad domains: richer relationships, an increased appreciation for life, changed life priorities and the perception of new possibilities, increased personal strength, and spiritual changes. PTG is similar to benefit-finding in response to trauma (Affleck & Tennen, 1996), but involves more pervasive cognitive and affective changes that occur within the individual. These changes are postulated to involve the breaking down and rebuilding of assumptions about life as a result of the trauma, rather than simply finding positivity in the face of adversity (Shand et al., 2015). To what extent and under what circumstances PTG occurs remains controversial. However, the concept of PTG has implications for understanding the development of human resilience and for the implementation of interventions such as Managing Cancer and Living Meaningfully (CALM) that support individuals facing the trauma of advanced cancer.

POSTTRAUMATIC GROWTH

PTG is assumed to result from confronting and successfully coping with trauma (Tedeschi & Calhoun, 1996). In advanced disease, this may occur when individuals learn to manage the psychological and physical burdens of disease, the loss of autonomy, and the threat of impending mortality. Fear, anxiety, and existential distress in this circumstance are difficult to face and manage, and doing so effectively is postulated to provide an opportunity for growth (Maxfield et al., 2013). Indeed, a growing body of research supports the view that successful coping with life-threatening illness may create opportunities for PTG (Barskova & Oesterreich, 2009; Maxfield et al., 2013).

MODELS OF POSTTRAUMATIC GROWTH

The notion that positive change can occur following traumatic events has been widely considered (Coyne & Tennen, 2010), and achieving this outcome is a goal of CALM. However, there is continued debate about whether PTG is an objectively real and observable outcome or is an illusory, but comforting, belief (Sumalla et al., 2009). In the following section, evidence is presented for each of these views in the context of advanced cancer.

Growth as Illusory

Two theories that conceptualize psychological growth following trauma as illusory are cognitive adaptation theory (Taylor, 1983) and temporal comparison theory of growth (Klauer et al., 1998). Both are built upon the premise that humans tend to cope with threat by relying on positive illusions and that growth depends on maintaining these positive illusions following a traumatic event. Cognitive adaptation theory further postulates that mastery or control over the trauma is achieved by ascribing positive meaning to an adverse event and by making downward comparisons with those who have fared less well (Taylor, 1983). Temporal comparison theory proposes that psychological equilibrium is maintained in response to current trauma by reframing past events as being more negative than they really were, supporting the view that things have now improved (Klauer et al., 1998). Both theories suggest that individuals rely on positive illusions of growth to cope with traumatic events and their aftermath, even when no real change has occurred in personal beliefs or world views. They propose instead that the apparent process of PTG is illusory, representing a form of defensive denial that serves to lower distress (Klauer et al., 1998).

A study conducted by Tallman and colleagues (2014) provides some empirical support for the view that PTG is a defensive strategy rather than an actual process of growth in individuals with advanced cancer. These authors found that cancer patients tended to overestimate the amount of growth that they had achieved, compared to estimates made by their family caregivers (Tallman et al., 2014). This tendency of patients to overestimate their growth may reflect the illusory nature of PTG and suggests that so-called growth may be a "biased means of self-preservation" (Tallman et al., 2014, p. 353). Whether this tendency to view oneself and one's life in a more positive way, even if not confirmed by external or objective criteria, is representative of growth is open to debate.

Growth as a Real Outcome

Contrasting the view that PTG is a self-protective illusion is the perspective that it reflects an actual, beneficial result of struggling with difficult circumstances. Three theoretical models adopt this view: the model of life crises (Schaefer & Moos, 1998), the organismic valuing theory (Joseph & Linley, 2005), and the model of world assumptions (Janoff-Bulman, 2006). In contrast to theories that regard growth as illusory, these models conceptualize growth as a real outcome that is shaped by the social context and personal resources of those affected.

The model of life crises postulates that heightened mortality salience following trauma prompts individuals to re-examine their values and needs. This re-examination may result in positive changes, such as seeking closer relationships or making greater use of social or personal resources (Schaefer & Moos, 1998). Similarly, organismic valuing theory posits that "people constantly evaluate whether their current experiences and actions are fulfilling their needs" (Joseph & Linley, 2005). Such constant evaluation is thought to change world schemes when there is discordance between current circumstances and the individual's basic psychological needs for autonomy, competence, and relatedness (Joseph & Linley, 2005). Thus, after trauma, individuals may shift their priorities to appreciate the positive aspects of their relationships or their circumstances and may be less bothered by more minor frustrations or disappointments.

The world assumptions model postulates that negative life events shatter basic assumptions, requiring the creation of a "new, non-threatening assumptive world" (Janoff-Bulman, 1992, p. 117). In this model, successful coping derives from a changed world scheme and is associated with an increased appreciation for life and changed life priorities. This model incorporates individual factors, such as optimism, that assist or impede growth (Schaefer & Moos, 1998).

Two studies of cancer patients and their caregivers provide evidence to support the notion that PTG is a real phenomenon. One is a study of breast cancer patients and their husbands (Weiss, 2002) and the other, of hepatobiliary cancer patients and their caregivers (Moore et al., 2011). Measures of growth were administered to patients and their loved ones in both studies, and loved ones were asked to report the growth that they perceived in the patient and in themselves. Both studies found that patients and their loved ones reported similar levels of growth, with moderate to high agreement between growth reported by patients and ratings of patient growth by caregivers. In addition, in a qualitative study of the growth experience in patients with head and neck cancer and their spouses, Ruf and colleagues (2009) found that patients and spouses reported similar levels of personal growth in the patient. These findings contrast with those of Tallman and colleagues (2014) and support the view that growth is a real outcome following traumatic events, rather than an illusory coping mechanism.

Growth as Both Real and Illusory

The final set of models do not place growth firmly in either the real or illusory category, suggesting instead that it can be both. The Janus-Face model (Maercker & Zoellner, 2004), the affective-cognitive process model (Joseph et al., 2012), and the functional-descriptive model of growth (Tedeschi & Calhoun, 1996, 2004) view growth as a multifaceted phenomenon that is, at times, both a real outcome and an illusory coping process.

The Janus-Face model (Maercker & Zoellner, 2004) is the most explicit in its definition of growth as neither illusory or real. Growth is characterized in this model as having two sides, much like the two faces of the mythical Roman god, Janus. There is the self-deceptive side, similar to that outlined in the cognitive affective model (Taylor, 1983), and a more functional, self-transcending side, as suggested by Schaefer and Moos (1998). Similarly, the affective-cognitive processing model considers growth to be simultaneously illusory and representative of actual psychological well-being (Joseph et al., 2012). The Janus-Face model considers the self-deceptive facet of growth to be a short-term coping mechanism, with real growth occurring over a longer period of time (Maercker & Zoellner, 2004). The affective-cognitive model proposes a curvilinear relationship between posttraumatic stress and PTG (Joseph et al., 2012). Both models concede that growth can be both illusory and real but disagree on the circumstances that favor one type over the other.

Finally, in an extension of the world assumptions model (Janoff-Bulman, 1992), the functional-descriptive model of growth (Tedeschi & Calhoun, 1996, 2004) purports that the discordance between previously held beliefs and those that occur following trauma prompts active rumination and attempts to restructure one's schema of the self and the world to achieve coherence in beliefs. This is highly relevant to the context of advanced disease, where the assumptions upon which individuals have based their lives may be undermined. As Tedeschi and Calhoun (2004) suggest, there may be dramatic alterations in one's sense of self, one's life philosophy, and one's relationships following trauma. CALM can be a powerful facilitator of change and growth in this situation.

POSTTRAUMATIC GROWTH AND CANCER

Tedeschi and Calhoun's (1996, 2004) five-component functional-descriptive model of growth is currently one of the most widely used in cancer research. However, Sumalla and colleagues (2009) have noted that PTG may interact with cancer in a way that differs from more discrete life-threatening events. The experience of advanced cancer is usually complex, with multiple stressful events that occur over a prolonged period of time. Additionally, cancer arises within the individual, making it more challenging to ignore or forget the signs of disease. The ability to sustain "double awareness" (Rodin & Zimmermann, 2008), in which distressing thoughts about traumatic events are balanced by other views, may be difficult for the cancer patient and could limit the potential for PTG.

MEASURING POSTTRAUMATIC GROWTH

Two standardized and validated scales have been widely used to measure PTG. These are the Post-Traumatic Growth Inventory (PTGI; Tedeschi &

Calhoun, 1996) and the Stress-Related Growth Scale (Park et al., 1996), with most quantitative studies in cancer relying on the former. In accordance with Tedeschi and Calhoun's model of growth, the PTGI is divided into five subscales: relating to others, new possibilities, personal strength, spiritual change, and appreciation for life. However, concerns have been raised regarding the validity of these subscales, the lack of consensus on the definitions of "trauma" and "growth," and the retrospective and self-report nature of both instruments (Bitsch et al., 2011). Furthermore, the PTGI items are phrased in a way that favors growth as an outcome instead of a process (e.g., "I established a new path for my life" rather than "I am establishing a new path for my life").

THE CLINICAL PROCESS

CALM was developed not only to relieve distress in patients with advanced disease but also to help them reconfigure their lives and relationships under the new circumstances into which they have been thrust. The latter is consistent with the concept of facing and adapting to challenging or traumatic circumstances that is central in theories of post-traumatic growth (Calhoun & Tedeschi, 2006). A new capacity to face fears related to the end of life may also be viewed as a manifestation of PTG, although this has not often been considered. Being able to shift world views in the aftermath of trauma may make individuals more resilient or resistant to subsequent distressing events (Janoff-Bulman, 2006).

Trauma not only can lead to disruption in relationships but can also result in a new or renewed sense of intimacy and closeness. As one patient enrolled in CALM said, "I'm groggy and I open my eyes and I see coming through the door, my wife and kids. There was this overwhelming feeling of love. It seemed as if my heart would overflow. Thinking that was a feeling that you have to, I think, be very lucky to experience." This same patient also reported seeing humanity as a whole and their medical caregivers in a new and meaningful way, saying, "You neglect to see the beautiful people that are around you, the ones who feel, who have compassion, who do things to help others. In a way, my experience with the radiation people and then with the chemotherapy people, I mean these people are such wonderful, wonderful human beings." And later, "Not only do I recognize the greater depth of feeling towards my own personal relationships but also towards humanity as a whole, if you want to put it that way, and more conscious of our responsibility towards one another." Another patient enrolled in CALM said, "I have to prepare myself for death, and she [the therapist] is managing to [help me] because feeling that I'm able to grow as a person makes me feel like I will be able to handle death in a peaceful way."

The flux that advanced cancer creates in the lives of those affected is reflected in the encounter of the patient with the CALM therapist. Both face the uncertainty and inevitability of the disease and question how the therapeutic encounter will unfold. At first, talk may seem like a weapon or tool not strong enough to overcome the devastation produced by advanced cancer. However, research has suggested a link between reflection and growth. Deliberate rumination or reflectiveness was positively associated with growth in a sample of cancer survivors, while intrusive rumination or brooding was associated with distress (Morris & Shakespeare-Finch, 2011). Similarly, instrumental rumination or reflection was positively associated with reports of PTG among women newly diagnosed with breast cancer (Soo & Sherman, 2015). More negatively oriented rumination (e.g., brooding or unintentional, intrusive rumination) is also associated with some components of PTG, perhaps representing cognitive attempts to process and cope with the trauma (Soo & Sherman, 2015). Determining the link between cognition and growth merits further investigation, but the evidence to date points to the potential therapeutic value of cognition in promoting growth. By providing reflective space and an opportunity for patients to consider their disease, its impact on their life, and the ways in which they can begin adjusting to an uncertain future, CALM opens up the possibility of growth. In the "now moment" (Stern et al., 1998) of the disease, all the assumptions that have guided the patient in their life and the therapist in their work are thrown up into the air. It is in this open field that a creative therapeutic process may emerge and in which PTG may occur.

CONCLUSION

The experience of positive growth as a result of coping with a life-threatening illness is an appealing notion for patients with advanced cancer. Whether PTG is a real, observable phenomenon or an illusory coping process continues to be a subject of debate. However, evidence suggests that PTG may occur in the context of advanced cancer when patients are able to master or accept the challenges of the disease and the distressing emotions that it evokes. By providing an open space for reflection and allowing patients to confront their new reality, CALM opens the possibility of growth at the end of life.

REFERENCES

Affleck, G., & Tennen, H. (1996). Construing benefits from adversity: Adaptational significance and dispositional underpinnings. *Journal of Personality, 64*(4), 899–922.

Barskova, T., & Oesterreich, R. (2009). Post-traumatic growth in people living with a serious medical condition and its relations to physical and mental health: A systematic review. *Disability and Rehabilitation, 31*(21), 1709–1733.

Bitsch, L. J., Elklit, A., & Christiansen, D. M. (2011). *Basic problems with the measurement of posttraumatic growth.* (Unpublished working paper). University of Southern Denmark.

Calhoun, L. G., & Tedeschi, R. G. (2006). The foundations of posttraumatic growth: An expanded framework. In L. G. Calhoun & R. G. Tedeschi (Eds.), *Handbook of posttraumatic growth: Research and practice,* (p. 3–23). New York, NY: Routledge.

Coyne, J. C., & Tennen, H. (2010). Positive psychology in cancer care: Bad science, exaggerated claims, and unproven medicine. *Annals of Behavioral Medicine, 39*(1), 16–26.

Janoff-Bulman, R. (1992). *Shattered assumptions: Towards a new psychology of trauma.* Free Press.

Janoff-Bulman, R. (2006). Schema-change perspectives on posttraumatic growth. In L. G. Calhoun & R. G. Tedeschi (Eds.), *Handbook of posttraumatic growth: Research and practice* (pp. 81–99). Routledge.

Joseph, S., & Linley, P. A. (2005). Positive adjustment to threatening events: An organismic valuing theory of growth through adversity. *Review of General Psychology, 9*(3), 262–280.

Joseph, S., Murphy, D., & Regel, S. (2012). An affective-cognitive processing model of post-traumatic growth. *Clinical Psychology & Psychotherapy, 19*(4), 316–325.

Klauer, T., Ferring, D., & Filipp, S. H. (1998). "Still stable after all this. . . .?": Temporal comparison in coping with severe and chronic disease. *International Journal of Behavioral Development, 22*(2), 339–355.

Maercker, A., & Zoellner, T. (2004). The Janus Face of self-perceived growth: Toward a two-component model of posttraumatic growth. *Psychological Inquiry, 15*(1), 41–48.

Maxfield, M., Pyszczynski, T., & Solomon, S. (2013). Finding meaning in death: Terror management among the terminally ill. In N. Straker (Ed.), *Facing cancer and the fear of death: A psychoanalytic perspective on treatment* (pp. 41–60). Jason Aronson.

Moore, A. M., Gamblin, T. C., Geller, D. A., Youssef, M. N., Hoffman, K. E., Gemmell, L., Likumahuwa, S. M., Bovbjerg, D. H., Marsland, A., & Steel, J. L. (2011). A prospective study of posttraumatic growth as assessed by self-report and family caregiver in the context of advanced cancer. *Psycho-Oncology, 20*(5), 479–487.

Morris, B. A., & Shakespeare-Finch, J. (2011). Rumination, post-traumatic growth, and distress: Structural equation modelling with cancer survivors. *Psycho-Oncology, 20*(11), 1176–1183.

Park, C. L., Cohen, L. H., & Murch, R. L. (1996). Assessment and prediction of stress-related growth. *Journal of Personality, 64*(1), 71–105.

Rodin, G., & Zimmermann, C. (2008). Psychoanalytic reflections on mortality: A reconsideration. *Journal of the American Academy of Psychoanalysis and Dynamic Psychiatry, 36*(1), 181–196.

Ruf, M., Büchi, S., Moergeli, H., Zwahlen, R. A., & Jenewein, J. (2009). Positive personal changes in the aftermath of head and neck cancer diagnosis: A qualitative study in patients and their spouses. *Head & Neck, 31*(4), 513–520.

Schaefer, J. A., & Moos, R. H. (1998). The context for posttraumatic growth: Life crises, individual and social resources, and coping. In R. G. Tedeschi, C. L. Park, & L. G. Calhoun (Eds.), *Posttraumatic growth: Positive changes in the aftermath of crisis* (pp. 99–125). Lawrence Erlbaum.

Shand, L. K., Cowlishaw, S., Brooker, J. E., Burney, S., & Ricciardelli, L. A. (2015). Correlates of post-traumatic stress symptoms and growth in cancer patients: A systematic review and meta-analysis. *Psycho-Oncology, 24*(6), 624–634.

Soo, H., & Sherman, K. A. (2015). Rumination, psychological distress and post-traumatic growth in women diagnosed with breast cancer. *Psycho-Oncology, 24*(1), 70–79.

Stern, D. N., Sander, L. W., Nahum, J. P., Harrison, A. M., Lyons-Ruth, K., Morgan, A. C., Bruschweiler-Stern, N., & Tronick, E. Z. (1998). Non-interpretive mechanisms in psychoanalytic therapy: The 'something more' than interpretation. *International Journal of Psycho-Analysis, 79,* (Pt 5) 903–921.

Sumalla, E. C., Ochoa, C., & Blanco, I. (2009). Posttraumatic growth in cancer: Reality or illusion? *Clinical Psychology Review, 29*(1), 24–33.

Tallman, B. A., Lohnberg, J., Yamada, T. H., Halfdanarson, T. R., & Altmaier, E. M. (2014). Anticipating posttraumatic growth from cancer: Patients' and collaterals' experiences. *Journal of Psychosocial Oncology, 32*(3), 342–358.

Taylor, S. E. (1983). Adjustment to threatening events: A theory of cognitive adaptation. *American Psychologist, 38*(11), 1161–1173.

Tedeschi, R., G. & Calhoun, L. G. (1996). The Posttraumatic Growth Inventory: Measuring the positive legacy of trauma. *Journal of Traumatic Stress, 9*(3), 455–471.

Tedeschi, R., G. & Calhoun, L. G. (2004). Posttraumatic growth: Conceptual foundations and empirical evidence. *Psychological Inquiry, 15*(1), 1–18.

Weiss, T. (2002). Posttraumatic growth in women with breast cancer and their husbands: An intersubjective validation study. *Journal of Psychosocial Oncology, 20*(2), 65–80.

Zoellner, T., & Maercker, A. (2006). Posttraumatic growth in clinical psychology—A critical review and introduction of a two component model. *Clinical Psychology Review, 26*(5), 626–653.

CHAPTER 9
The Context of CALM

[T]he best part of being able to come here and talk to somebody [is] that I can kind of . . . share my fears and not feel like I'm burdening this other person with all this terrible, terrible information.
—CALM participant

WHY CALM?

The findings of the Will to Live study that depression and demoralization are common in patients with advanced disease and grow worse toward the end of life in the absence of any intervention convinced us that something must be done to prevent this outcome (see Chapter 3 of this volume). We looked for an evidence-based intervention appropriate for both individuals and couples that was focused as much on helping those with advanced disease live as meaningfully as possible as it was on relieving their distress. Although groundbreaking work had been done on the psychological treatment of patients with advanced disease, much of it had been tailored to groups (e.g., Spiegel et al., 1981, 1999; Breitbart et al., 2015; Kissane et al., 2007). We could not find a meaningful and appropriate intervention designed specifically for individuals and couples living with advanced disease that was integrated into cancer care and palliative care. Building on the work of others in group therapy and on our own clinical experience, theoretical background, and research, we proceeded to develop CALM. We felt committed to ensuring that benefit would accrue from the generosity of the many patients who had participated in our research over the past two decades and were compelled to improve care for the generations of patients to follow. It was also not coincidental that our work emerged as part of a broader interest in early palliative care, both at our center and beyond.

EARLY AND LATE PALLIATIVE CARE

Palliative care has existed in one form or another since antiquity, although the modern field of palliative care is little more than 50 years old. Its birth is often marked by the opening of St. Christopher's Hospice in London, England, guided by the pioneering leadership of Dame Cicely Saunders in holistic end-of-life care. Perhaps equally important in drawing attention to the needs of individuals and their families facing the end of life was Elisabeth Kübler-Ross, a Swiss psychiatrist who emigrated to America, where she began to work with dying patients. Challenging the taboo about open conversation regarding the end of life that existed in medicine and in broader society at that time, she was one of the first to demonstrate that dying patients can be helped by contemplating and talking about death. Her 1969 seminal book, *On Death and Dying* (Kübler-Ross, 1969; see Chapter 3 of this volume), was transformative in ending the conspiracy of silence around those who were dying. However, it was Balfour Mount, a Canadian surgeon who studied with Kübler-Ross in England, who coined the term "palliative care" to avoid the stigma associated with the term "hospice." It was not until several decades later that palliative care came to be defined as the psychological, social, and spiritual care of patients and families from the time of diagnosis of a life-threatening disease (World Health Organization, 1990). A large body of research has since demonstrated the benefit of early palliative care on the quality of life and well-being of patients with advanced cancer (Temel et al., 2010; Zimmermann et al., 2014).

The growth of research and clinical services in palliative care in recent decades has been remarkable, but there has been a greater focus in the field on managing pain and physical symptoms than on managing psychological distress. The relative lack of systematic approaches to the psychological care of patients with advanced disease is striking, given that psychological distress is often the most prominent symptom at early stages of disease (see Chapter 2 of this volume). This prioritization of the body over the mind reflects an overarching tendency in modern medicine to regard interventions that involve empathy—perhaps the least expensive of all medical interventions—less highly than those that involve biology and technology (Napier et al., 2014; Rodin, An, et al., 2020). The introduction of CALM is an attempt to fill the gap that has existed in the psychological dimensions of early palliative care. CALM was developed to provide a framework for the content and process of the psychological care of patients living with advanced disease. This chapter highlights the relationship of CALM to earlier interventions and to its integration with cancer care and palliative care.

INTERVENTIONS FOR DISTRESS AT THE ONSET OF LIFE-THREATENING OR ADVANCED CANCER

Many patients with advanced cancer in high-income countries are now re- ferred to palliative care early in the course of their disease (Watson et al., 2018), but most do not receive specialized or tailored psychological care (Institute of Medicine, 2008; Li et al., 2017). This lack of specialized psy- chological care persists despite the overwhelming fear and anxiety that individuals experience early in the disease trajectory and the difficulties they may have in understanding their illness and what it means for them (see Chapter 2 of this volume). Specialized psychosocial care may need to be embedded in the cancer treatment setting for it to be implemented in a timely and routine fashion without stigmatization.

Recent research on the immediate psychological impact of the diag- nosis, recurrence, or progression of advanced or life-threatening cancer has shown that traumatic stress symptoms, which may meet criteria for acute stress disorder or posttraumatic stress disorder, are common at such times (see Chapter 2 of this volume). Our research has demonstrated that one third of patients diagnosed with acute leukemia experience traumatic stress symptoms that meet criteria for threshold or subthreshold acute stress disorder (Rodin et al., 2013; see Chapter 2 of this volume). These traumatic stress symptoms persisted or recurred in over half of individuals in the three months following diagnosis (Rodin et al., 2018) and were as- sociated with substantial physical symptom burden (Zimmermann et al., 2013). To treat and prevent these manifestations of physical and psycho- logical distress, we developed an intervention referred to as Emotion And Symptom-focused Engagement (EASE; Rodin, Malfitano, et al., 2020). EASE has some features in common with CALM but also includes specific techniques to manage the anxiety and posttraumatic stress symptoms that are prevalent early in the course of the disease. EASE is integrated with a triggered palliative symptom control intervention. A recent phase II randomized controlled trial (RCT) demonstrated the feasibility of EASE and found significant improvements in traumatic stress symptoms and in the intensity and management of pain (Rodin, Malfitano, et al., 2020). We are now conducting a multisite randomized clinical trial to confirm the effectiveness of this intervention.

Two other pilot RCTs of interventions designed for recently diagnosed patients with advanced cancer have reported encouraging findings. The first, a one- to four-session supportive-expressive meaning-making intervention, was shown to improve meaning and existential well-being in patients with advanced ovarian cancer when compared to usual care (Henry et al., 2010). The other, a six-session multidisciplinary intervention, found a positive effect on quality of life for a mixed group of patients with advanced cancer receiving radiotherapy when compared to usual care (Clark et al., 2013). The latter intervention included conditioning and relaxation exercises, education, cognitive behavioral strategies for coping with cancer, and open discussion and support.

INTERVENTIONS FOR THOSE LIVING WITH METASTATIC AND ADVANCED CANCER

Many psychotherapeutic interventions for metastatic cancer include elements of supportive-expressive therapy. Hallmarks of these interventions include the establishment of a relationship in which there is a conversation over time, emotional support, modulation of affect, and a shared task of finding meaning and facing relevant problems (Rodin, An, et al., 2020). David Spiegel and his group at Stanford found that supportive-expressive group therapy allowed women with metastatic breast cancer to feel supported, express disease-related emotions, and face existential concerns (Classen et al., 2001). RCTs of this group intervention, which consisted of weekly open-ended sessions over 8 to 12 months led by psychiatrists, social workers, psychologists, or nurses, demonstrated that it could also improve mood (Classen et al., 2001; Goodwin et al., 2001), emotional control and coping (Giese-Davis et al., 2002), and reduce traumatic stress symptoms in women with metastatic breast cancer (Classen et al., 2001; Kissane et al., 2007). However, the frequency and duration of the sessions and the geographic distance of participants from treatment settings posed challenges for the routine integration of the intervention. For this reason, a version of the therapy delivered via teleconference was developed, and preliminary results have shown it to be feasible and acceptable (O'Brien et al., 2008).

We have similarly found that patients suffering from significant burden of disease who must balance many scheduled clinic appointments, tests, and interventions are often unable to attend group therapy sessions at a fixed time. Further, many of these individuals are unable to absorb the distress of others in the group when they are struggling to manage their own. They typically want a private place to discuss their own personal and family concerns. Group therapy is not usually feasible or desired in this circumstance, although it may be appropriate with more chronic disease.

Meaning-centered approaches, in which enhancing meaning is the main therapeutic aim (Vos & Vitali, 2018), have frequently been employed with patients living with advanced cancer, and a growing body of evidence supports their value. The most well-known is meaning-centered psychotherapy (MCP), developed by Breitbart and colleagues (2015). MCP is a brief, manualized intervention tailored to individuals living with advanced cancer. Rooted in the therapeutic framework of Viktor Frankl's logotherapy (Frankl, 1988), MCP is designed to help patients with advanced cancer sustain or enhance a sense of meaning, peace, and purpose (Breitbart et al., 2010). It was originally designed as an eight-session group intervention that included psychoeducation on the concepts of meaning, peace, and purpose, which was further enhanced by experiential exercises and group discussions. In a large RCT, MCP was found to significantly improve spiritual well-being, quality of life, and depression compared to a manualized supportive group psychotherapy intervention (Breitbart et al., 2015). However, because of the logistical challenges for patients with metastatic cancer to attend the fixed scheduled times of group sessions, an individualized version of MCP (IMCP) was developed and tested. An RCT evaluating its effectiveness showed significant effects for IMCP on quality of life, sense of meaning, and spiritual well-being compared to usual care (Breitbart et al., 2018). The focus on the sense of meaning and purpose in MCP overlaps with one of the domains of CALM and with its overall intent.

Cognitive behavioral therapies (CBTs) have also been utilized in patients with advanced cancer. These psychological interventions were developed to shape meaning and behavior and aim to reduce emotional distress by identifying, analyzing, and modifying dysfunctional or distorted thoughts or behavior (Beck et al., 1985). A modified CBT focusing on clinically relevant problems and thoughts that may be rational but are intrusive, such as those related to pain, disability, and death (Greer et al., 2010; Moorey & Greer, 2002), has been recommended for application in advanced cancer. Some pilot studies indicate that a cognitive-behavioral approach might reduce anxiety in patients with advanced disease (Greer et al., 2012; Moorey et al., 2009), but the impact of CBT on depression in advanced cancer has been more variable. Two RCTs evaluating brief CBT interventions in patients with metastatic breast cancer demonstrated significant reductions in depressive symptoms immediately postintervention (Edelman et al., 1999) and at six-month follow-up (Savard et al., 2006). However, another evaluating CBT delivered by trained home palliative care nurses in an advanced cancer population failed to show reductions in depressive symptoms (Moorey et al., 2009). Most recently, a large RCT evaluating the impact of a manualized CBT on depression and other secondary outcomes in advanced cancer outpatients recruited from primary care, oncology, or hospices did not find it to be effective (Serfaty et al., 2019).

There are other promising interventions developed and evaluated for use in advanced cancer, including collaborative care models for treating depression (e.g., Sharpe et al., 2014), mindfulness-based interventions (e.g., Chambers et al., 2017; Foley et al., 2010; Schellekens et al., 2017; Zimmermann et al., 2018), and couple-based interventions (e.g., Kuijer et al., 2004; McLean et al., 2013; Northouse et al., 2013). Team-based collaborative care involving cancer nurses, consultation-liaison psychiatrists, and primary care physicians was found to be more effective than usual care in the treatment of depression in patients with lung cancer (Walker et al., 2014). Other interventions that have shown promise include family-based grief therapy (e.g., Kissane et al., 2006, 2016) and structured psychotherapy for older adults with advanced disease (e.g., Mantovani et al., 1996a, 1996b).

INTERVENTIONS NEAR THE END OF LIFE

A number of interventions have been developed for individuals with advanced cancer nearing the end of life. These include Dignity Therapy (Chochinov et al., 2005), short-term life review (Ando et al., 2008), and narrative interventions (Lloyd-Williams et al., 2018; Wise et al., 2018). These interventions are designed to be brief and involve individualized interviews that aim to engender a sense of meaning and purpose through life review. Participants are asked questions such as "What is the most important thing in your life and why?" (Ando et al., 2010), "What are your most important accomplishments?" (Chochinov et al., 2005), and "What would you want your family, friends, or loved ones to remember about you?" (Wise et al., 2018). The interview is then transcribed and edited into a generativity/legacy document (Dignity Therapy), a collage album (short-term life review), or a life story (Wise et al., 2018), which is reviewed by the patient. The final document is left with the patient to pass on to their family or close others as they wish. Of these, Dignity Therapy has been the most widely studied.

The initial pilot feasibility study of Dignity Therapy conducted by Chochinov and colleagues (2005) reported significant improvements in suffering and depressive symptoms in Canadian and Australian samples. High levels of acceptability and satisfaction with Dignity Therapy have also been shown (Fitchett et al., 2015), although a subsequent multisite RCT conducted in Canada, Australia, and the United States did not confirm its effect on distress (Chochinov et al., 2011). Other research from the United Kingdom, Portugal, and Denmark has been similarly inconsistent with regard to the efficacy of the intervention in reducing distress (Hall et al., 2011, 2012; Houmann et al., 2014; Julião et al., 2014). However, Dignity Therapy has been shown to create and/or enhance the sense of legacy and meaning for many patients (Chochinov et al., 2011).

BARRIERS TO THE OPTIMAL DELIVERY OF PSYCHOLOGICAL CARE

Some of the challenges to the delivery of CALM are common to all psychological interventions with advanced disease. A core group of trained health-care providers is required in oncology and palliative care settings to deliver specialized interventions of this kind, to train other health professionals in their delivery, and to ensure ongoing treatment integrity. At present, the breadth and depth of these resources in cancer treatment centers are highly variable. Advocacy is needed to heighten awareness of clinicians and policymakers of the potential benefit of specialized psychosocial interventions in oncology and palliative care and of the need to allocate resources for their delivery.

Measuring outcomes with psychological interventions is extremely important both to establish their effectiveness and to monitor their quality. Psychological outcome measures that were developed for other populations may not be valid or reliable in patients with advanced disease (Kelly et al., 2006). The modification, development, and validation of psychometric tools for patients with advanced disease has improved the quality of research on psychological interventions in palliative care. These newer tools include the Demoralization Scale-II (Robinson et al., 2016), the Schedule of Attitudes Toward Hastened Death (Rosenfeld et al., 1999), the Death and Dying Distress Scale (Krause et al., 2015), the Quality of Dying and Death Questionnaire (Mah et al., 2019; Patrick et al., 2001), and the Experiences in Close Relationships scale (Lo et al., 2009). We specifically developed the Clinical Evaluation Questionnaire (Lo et al., 2015; de Vries et al., 2020) to assess the perceived benefit of

CALM three and six months after initiation of therapy (see Chapter 10 of this volume). This measure is intended to evaluate the process of CALM and guide therapeutic intervention. The availability of relevant psychometric tools has added rigor to the assessment of outcomes of psychological interventions in palliative care, to the supervision of therapists, to the evaluation of treatment integrity, and to the assessment of the quality of clinical care.

Distress screening has been recommended as a standard of cancer care and has been successfully implemented in multiple cancer centers to identify patients with elevated distress levels who can then be assessed and referred, as needed, for specialized psychosocial care (Li et al., 2016; Zebrack et al., 2015). Such measures may be most efficiently completed electronically with intelligent programming, allowing scores on single items to trigger the completion of additional specific validated measures (Bagha et al., 2013). Screening for distress in patients with advanced cancer and their primary caregivers may help identify those in most urgent need of specialized psychosocial care, although its value depends on timely referral and access to care. While many cancer settings have distress screening protocols, adherence and responsiveness to them are inconsistent (Zebrack et al., 2017), and the allocation of resources to provide appropriate psychosocial care is insufficient in many settings.

CONCLUSION

CALM builds on a foundation of work in the psychotherapeutic treatment of patients with advanced disease. These include interventions at the time of diagnosis, in which there is a focus on anxiety and posttraumatic stress symptoms; those implemented during the course of the disease, in which there is often a focus on a sense of meaning in life; and those provided at the end of life, in which there is particular attention to the sense of legacy. The scientific rigor of research investigating the impact of these interventions in palliative care has improved dramatically over the past decade, largely due to the availability of relevant, validated measures to assess outcomes. Further investigation is required to determine the subgroups most likely to respond to specific interventions; the generalizability of the findings; and the relevance, acceptability, and feasibility of interventions in diverse regional, cultural, and religious settings. Implementation science methodologies (Proctor et al., 2009) are now being employed to identify optimal strategies of integration for psychosocial interventions with global oncology and palliative care.

REFERENCES

Ando, M., Morita, T., Akechi, T., Okamoto, T., & Japanese Task Force for Spiritual Care. (2010). Efficacy of short-term life-review interviews on the spiritual well-being of terminally ill cancer patients. *Journal of Pain and Symptom Management, 39*(6), 993–1002.

Ando, M., Morita, T., Okamoto, T., & Ninosaka, Y. (2008). One-week short-term life review interview can improve spiritual well-being of terminally ill cancer patients. *Psycho-Oncology, 17*(9), 885–890.

Bagha, S. M., Macedo, A., Jacks, L. M., Lo, C., Zimmermann, C., Rodin, G., & Li, M. (2013). The utility of the Edmonton Symptom Assessment System in screening for anxiety and depression. *European Journal of Cancer Care, 22*(1), 60–69.

Beck, A., Emery, G., & Greenberg, R. L. (1985). *Anxiety disorders and phobias. A cognitive perspective.* Basic Books.

Breitbart, W., Pessin, H., Rosenfeld, B., Applebaum, A. J., Lichtenthal, W. G., Li, Y., Saracino, R. M., Marziliano, A. M., Masterson, M., Tobias, K., & Fenn, N. (2018). Individual meaning-centered psychotherapy for the treatment of psychological and existential distress: A randomized controlled trial in patients with advanced cancer. *Cancer, 124*(15), 3231–3239.

Breitbart, W., Rosenfeld, B., Gibson, C., Pessin, H., Poppito, S., Nelson, C., Tomarken, A., Timm, A.K., Berg, A., Jacobson, C., Sorger, B., Abbey, J., & Olden, M. (2010). Meaning-centered group psychotherapy for patients with advanced cancer: A pilot randomized controlled trial. *Psycho-Oncology, 19*(1), 21–28.

Breitbart, W., Rosenfeld, B., Pessin, H., Applebaum, A., Kulikowski, J., & Lichtenthal, W. G. (2015). Meaning-centered group psychotherapy: An effective intervention for improving psychological well-being in patients with advanced cancer. *Journal of Clinical Oncology, 33*(7), 749–754.

Chambers, S. K., Occhipinti, S., Foley, E., Clutton, S., Legg, M., Berry, M., Stockler, M. R., Frydenberg, M., Gardiner, R. A., Lepore, S. J., Davis, I. D., & Smith, D. P. (2017). Mindfulness-based cognitive therapy in advanced prostate cancer: A randomized controlled trial. *Journal of Clinical Oncology, 35*(3), 291–297.

Chochinov, H. M., Hack, T., Hassard, T., Kristjanson, L. J., McClement, S., & Harlos, M. (2005). Dignity therapy: A novel psychotherapeutic intervention for patients near the end of life. *Journal of Clinical Oncology, 23*(24), 5520–5525.

Chochinov, H. M., Kristjanson, L. J., Breitbart, W., McClement, S., Hack, T. F., Hassard, T., & Harlos, M. (2011). Effect of dignity therapy on distress and end-of-life experience in terminally ill patients: A randomised controlled trial. *The Lancet Oncology, 12*(8), 753–762.

Clark, M. M., Rummans, T. A., Atherton, P. J., Cheville, A. L., Johnson, M. E., Frost, M. H., Miller, J. J., Sloan, J. A., Graszer, K. M., Haas, J. G., Hanson, J. M., Garces, Y. I., Piderman, K. M., Lapid, M. I., Netzel, P. J., Richardson, J. W., & Brown, P. D. (2013). Randomized controlled trial of maintaining quality of life during radiotherapy for advanced cancer. *Cancer, 119*(4), 880–887.

Classen, C., Butler, L. D., Koopman, C., Miller, E., DiMiceli, S., Giese-Davis, J., Fobair, P., Carlson, R.W., Kraemer, H.C., & Spiegel, D. (2001). Supportive-expressive group therapy and distress in patients with metastatic breast cancer: A randomized clinical intervention trial. *Archives of General Psychiatry, 58*(5), 494–501.

de Vries, F. E., Mah, K., Shapiro, G., Rydall, A., Hales, S., & Rodin, G. (2020). Assessing the process of a brief psychotherapy for patients with advanced cancer. (Submitted for publication).

Edelman, S., Bell, D. R., & Kidman, A. D. (1999). A group cognitive behaviour therapy programme with metastatic breast cancer patients. *Psycho-Oncology, 8*(4), 295–305.

Fitchett, G., Emanuel, L., Handzo, G., Boyken, L., & Wilkie, D. J. (2015). Care of the human spirit and the role of dignity therapy: A systematic review of dignity therapy research. *BMC Palliative Care, 14, 8.* doi: 10.1186/s12904-015-0007-1.

Foley, E., Baillie, A., Huxter, M., Price, M., & Sinclair, E. (2010). Mindfulness-based cognitive therapy for individuals whose lives have been affected by cancer: A randomized controlled trial. *Journal of Consulting and Clinical Psychology, 78*(1), 72–79.

Frankl, V. E. (1988). *The will to meaning: Foundations and applications of logotherapy* (Rev. ed.). Meridian/Plume.

Giese-Davis, J., Koopman, C., Butler, L. D., Classen, C., Cordova, M., Fobair, P., Benson, J., Kraemer, H. C., & Spiegel, D. (2002). Change in emotion-regulation strategy for women with metastatic breast cancer following supportive-expressive group therapy. *Journal of Consulting and Clinical Psychology, 70*(4), 916–925.

Goodwin, P. J., Leszcz, M., Ennis, M., Koopmans, J., Vincent, L., Guther, H., Drysdale, E., Hundleby, M., Chochinov, H. M., Navarro, M., Speca, M., & Hunter, J. (2001). The effect of group psychosocial support on survival in metastatic breast cancer. *The New England Journal of Medicine, 345*(24), 1719–1726.

Greer, J. A., Park, E. R., Prigerson, H. G., & Safren, S. A. (2010). Tailoring cognitive-behavioral therapy to treat anxiety comorbid with advanced cancer. *Journal of Cognitive Psychotherapy, 24*(4), 294–313.

Greer, J. A., Traeger, L., Bemis, H., Solis, J., Hendriksen, E. S., Park, E. R., Pirl, W. F., Temel, J. S., Prigerson, H. G., & Safren, S. A. (2012). A pilot randomized controlled trial of brief cognitive-behavioral therapy for anxiety in patients with terminal cancer. *The Oncologist, 17*(10), 1337–1345.

Hall, S., Goddard, C., Opio, D., Speck, P., & Higginson, I. J. (2012). Feasibility, acceptability and potential effectiveness of Dignity Therapy for older people in care homes: A phase II randomized controlled trial of a brief palliative care psychotherapy. *Palliative Medicine, 26*(5), 703–712.

Hall, S., Goddard, C., Opio, D., Speck, P. W., Martin, P., & Higginson, I. J. (2011). A novel approach to enhancing hope in patients with advanced cancer: A randomised phase II trial of dignity therapy. *BMJ Supportive & Palliative Care, 1*(3), 315–321.

Henry, M., Cohen, S. R., Lee, V., Sauthier, P., Provencher, D., Drouin, P., Gauthier, P., Gotlieb, W., Lau, S., Drummond, N., Gilbert, L., Stanimir, G., Sturgeon, J., Chasen, M., Mitchell, J., Huang, L. N., Ferland, M. K., & Mayo, N. (2010). The Meaning-Making intervention (MMi) appears to increase meaning in life in advanced ovarian cancer: A randomized controlled pilot study. *Psycho-Oncology, 19*(12), 1340–1347.

Houmann, L. J., Chochinov, H. M., Kristjanson, L. J., Petersen, M. A., & Groenvold, M. (2014). A prospective evaluation of Dignity Therapy in advanced cancer patients admitted to palliative care. *Palliative Medicine, 28*(5), 448–458.

Institute of Medicine (US) Committee on Psychosocial Services to Cancer Patients/ Families in a Community Setting. (2008). Cancer care for the whole patient: Meeting psychosocial health needs. Adler, N. E., Page, A. E .K., editors. National Academies Press (US). https://doi.org/10.17226/11993.

Julião, M., Oliveira, F., Nunes, B., Vaz Carneiro, A., & Barbosa, A. (2014). Efficacy of dignity therapy on depression and anxiety in Portuguese terminally ill patients: A phase II randomized controlled trial. *Journal of Palliative Medicine, 17*(6), 688–695.

Kelly, B., McClement, S., & Chochinov, H. M. (2006). Measurement of psychological distress in palliative care. *Palliative Medicine, 20*(8), 779–789.

Kissane, D. W., Grabsch, B., Clarke, D. M., Smith, G. C., Love, A. W., Bloch, S., Snyder, R.D., & Li, Y. (2007). Supportive-expressive group therapy for women with metastatic breast cancer: Survival and psychosocial outcome from a randomized controlled trial. *Psycho-Oncology, 16*(4), 277–286.

Kissane, D. W., McKenzie, M., Bloch, S., Moskowitz, C., McKenzie, D. P., & O'Neill, I. (2006). Family focused grief therapy: A randomized, controlled trial in palliative care and bereavement. *American Journal of Psychiatry, 163*(7), 1208–1218.

Kissane, D. W., Zaider, T. I., Li, Y., Hichenberg, S., Schuler, T., Lederberg, M., Lavelle, L., Loeb, R., & Del Gaudio, F. (2016). Randomized controlled trial of family therapy in advanced cancer continued into bereavement. *Journal of Clinical Oncology, 34*(16), 1921–1927.

Krause, S., Rydall, A., Hales, S., Rodin, G., & Lo, C. (2015). Initial validation of the Death and Dying Distress Scale for the assessment of death anxiety in patients with advanced cancer. *Journal of Pain and Symptom Management, 49*(1), 126–134.

Kübler-Ross, E. (1969). *On death and dying.* Tavistock Publications.

Kuijer, R. G., Buunk, B. P., De Jong, G. M., Ybema, J. F., & Sanderman, R. (2004). Effects of a brief intervention program for patients with cancer and their partners on feelings of inequity, relationship quality and psychological distress. *Psycho-Oncology, 13*(5), 321–334.

Li, M., Macedo, A., Crawford, S., Bagha, S., Leung, Y. W., Zimmermann, C., Fitzgerald, B., Wyatt, M., Stuart-McEwan, T., & Rodin, G. (2016). Easier said than done: Keys to successful implementation of the Distress Assessment and Response Tool (DART) program. *Journal of Oncology Practice, 12*(5), e513–e526. doi: 10.1200/JOP.2015.010066.

Li, M., Watt, S., Escaf, M., Gardam, M., Heesters, A., O'Leary, G., & Rodin, G. (2017). Medical assistance in dying—Implementing a hospital-based program in Canada. *The New England Journal of Medicine, 376*(21), 2082–2088.

Lloyd-Williams, M., Shiels, C., Ellis, J., Abba, K., Gaynor, E., Wilson, K., & Dowrick, C. (2018). Pilot randomised controlled trial of focused narrative intervention for moderate to severe depression in palliative care patients: DISCERN trial. *Palliative Medicine, 32*(1), 206–215.

Lo, C., Hales, S., Rydall, A., Panday, T., Chiu, A., Malfitano, C., Jung, J., Li, M., Nissim, R., Zimmermann. C., & Rodin, G. (2015). Managing Cancer And Living Meaningfully: Study protocol for a randomized controlled trial. *Trials*, 16, 391. doi: 10.1186/s13063-015-0811-1

Lo, C., Walsh, A., Mikulincer, M., Gagliese, L., Zimmermann, C., & Rodin, G. (2009). Measuring attachment security in patients with advanced cancer: Psychometric properties of a modified and brief Experiences in Close Relationships scale. *Psycho-Oncology, 18*(5), 490–499.

Mah, K., Hales, S., Weerakkody, I., Liu, L., Fernandes, S., Rydall, A., Vehling, S., Zimmermann, C., & Rodin, G. (2019). Measuring the quality of dying and death in advanced cancer: Item characteristics and factor structure of the Quality of Dying and Death Questionnaire. *Palliative Medicine, 33*(3), 369–380.

Mantovani, G., Astara, G., Lampis, B., Bianchi, A., Curreli, L., Orrù, W., Carta, M. G., Carpiniello, B., Contu, P., & Rudas, N. (1996a). Evaluation by multidimensional instruments of health-related quality of life of elderly cancer patients undergoing three different "psychosocial" treatment approaches. A randomized clinical trial. *Supportive Care in Cancer, 4*(2), 129–140.

Mantovani, G., Astara, G., Lampis, B., Bianchi, A., Curreli, L., Orrù, W., Carpiniello, B., Carta, M. G., Sorentino, M., & Rudas, N. (1996b). Impact of psychosocial intervention on the quality of life of elderly cancer patients. *Psycho-Oncology, 5*(2), 127–135.

McLean, L. M., Walton, T., Rodin, G., Esplen, M. J., & Jones, J. M. (2013). A couple-based intervention for patients and caregivers facing end-stage cancer: Outcomes of a randomized controlled trial. *Psycho-Oncology, 22*(1), 28–38.

Moorey, S., Cort, E., Kapari, M., Monroe, B., Hansford, P., Mannix, K., Henderson, M., Fisher, L., & Hotopf, M. (2009). A cluster randomized controlled trial of cognitive behaviour therapy for common mental disorders in patients with advanced cancer. *Psychological Medicine, 39*(5), 713–723.

Moorey, S., & Greer, S. (2002). *Cognitive behaviour therapy for people with cancer*. Oxford University Press.

Napier, A. D., Ancarno, C., Butler, B., Calabrese, J., Chater, A., Chatterjee, H., Guesnet, F., Horne, R., Jacyna, S., Jadhav, S., Macdonald, A., Neuendorf, U., Parkhurst, A., Reynolds, R., Scambler, G., Shamdasani, S., Smith, S. Z., Stougaard-Nielsen, J., Thomson, L., Tyler, N., Volkmann, A. M., Walker, T., Watson, J., Williams, A. C., Willott, C., Wilson, J., & Woolf, K. (2014). Culture and health. *The Lancet, 384*(9954), 1607–1639.

Northouse, L. L., Mood, D. W., Schafenacker, A., Kalemkerian, G., Zalupski, M., LoRusso, P., Hayes, D. F., Hussain, M., Ruckdeschel, J., Fendrick, A. M., Trask, P. C., Ronis, D. L., & Kershaw, T. (2013). Randomized clinical trial of a brief and extensive dyadic intervention for advanced cancer patients and their family caregivers. *Psycho-Oncology, 22*(3), 555–563.

O'Brien, M., Harris, J., King, R., & O'Brien, T. (2008). Supportive-expressive group therapy for women with metastatic breast cancer: Improving access for Australian women through use of teleconference. *Counselling and Psychotherapy Research, 8*(1), 28–35.

Patrick, D. L., Engelberg, R. A., & Curtis, J. R. (2001). Evaluating the quality of dying and death. *Journal of Pain and Symptom Management, 22*(3), 717–726.

Proctor, E. K., Landsverk, J., Aarons, G., Chambers, D., Glisson, C., & Mittman, B. (2009). Implementation research in mental health services: An emerging science with conceptual, methodological, and training challenges. *Administration and Policy in Mental Health and Mental Health Services Research, 36*(1), 24–34.

Robinson, S., Kissane, D. W., Brooker, J., Hempton, C., Michael, N., Fischer, J., Franco, M., Sulistio, M., Clarke, D. M., Ozmen, M., & Burney, S. (2016). Refinement and revalidation of the demoralization scale: The DS-II—External validity. *Cancer, 122*(14), 2260–2267.

Rodin, G., An, E., Shnall, J., & Malfitano, C. (2020). Psychological interventions for patients with advanced disease: Implications for oncology and palliative care. *Journal of Clinical Oncology, 38*(9), 885–904.

Rodin, G., Deckert, A., Tong, E., Le, L. W., Rydall, A., Schimmer, A., Marmar, C. R., Lo, C., & Zimmermann, C. (2018). Traumatic stress in patients with acute leukemia: A prospective cohort study. *Psycho-Oncology, 27*(2), 515–523.

Rodin, G., Malfitano, C., Rydall, A., Schimmer, A., Marmar, C. R., Mah, K., Lo, C., Nissim, R., & Zimmermann, C. (2020). Emotion And Symptom-focused Engagement (EASE): A randomized phase II trial of an integrated psychological and palliative care intervention for patients with acute leukemia. *Supportive Care in Cancer, 28*(1), 163–176.

Rodin, G., Yuen, D., Mischitelle, A., Minden, M. D., Brandwein, J., Schimmer, A., Marmar, C., Gagliese, L., Lo, C., Rydall, A., & Zimmermann, C. (2013). Traumatic stress in acute leukemia. *Psycho-Oncology, 22*(2), 299–307.

Rosenfeld, B., Breitbart, W., Stein, K., Funesti-Esch, J., Kaim, M., Krivo, S., & Galietta, M. (1999). Measuring desire for death among patients with HIV/AIDS: The Schedule of Attitudes Toward Hastened Death. *American Journal of Psychiatry, 156*(1), 94–100.

Savard, J., Simard, S., Giguère, I., Ivers, H., Morin, C. M., Maunsell, E., Gagnon, P., Robert, J., & Marceau, D. (2006). Randomized clinical trial on cognitive therapy for depression in women with metastatic breast cancer: Psychological and immunological effects. *Palliative & Supportive Care, 4*(3), 219–237.

Schellekens, M. P. J., van den Hurk, D. G. M., Prins, J. B., Donders, A. R.T., Molema, J., Dekhuijzen, R., van der Drift, M. A., & Speckens, A. E. M. (2017). Mindfulness-based stress reduction added to care as usual for lung cancer patients and/ or their partners: A multicentre randomized controlled trial. *Psycho-Oncology, 26*(12), 2118–2126.

Serfaty, M., King, M., Nazareth, I., Moorey, S., Aspden, T., Tookman, A., Mannix, K., Gola, A., Davis, S., Wood, J., Jones, L. (2019). Manualised cognitive behavioural therapy in treating depression in advanced cancer: The CanTalk RCT. *Health Technology Assessment, 23*(19), 1–106.

Sharpe, M., Walker, J., Hansen, C. H., Martin, P., Symeonides, S., Gourley, C., Wall, L., Weller, D., Murray, G., & SMaRT (Symptom Management Research Trials) Oncology-2 Team. (2014). Integrated collaborative care for comorbid major depression in patients with cancer (SMaRT Oncology-2): A multicentre randomised controlled effectiveness trial. *The Lancet, 384*(9948), 1099–1108.

Spiegel, D., Bloom, J. R., & Yalom, I. (1981). Group support for patients with metastatic cancer: A randomized outcome study. *Archives of General Psychiatry, 38*(5), 527–533.

Spiegel, D., Morrow, G. R., Classen, C., Raubertas, R., Stott, P. B., Mudaliar, N., Pierce, H. I., Flynn, P. J., Heard, L., & Riggs, G. (1999). Group psychotherapy for recently diagnosed breast cancer patients: A multicenter feasibility study. *Psycho-Oncology, 8*(6), 482–493.

Temel, J. S., Greer, J. A., Muzikansky, A., Gallagher, E. R., Admane, S., Jackson, V. A., Dahlin, C. M., Blinderman, C. D., Jacobsen, J., Pirl, W. F., Billings, J. A., & Lynch, T. J. (2010). Early palliative care for patients with metastatic non–small-cell lung cancer. *The New England Journal of Medicine, 363*(8), 733–742.

Vos, J., & Vitali, D. (2018). The effects of psychological meaning-centered therapies on quality of life and psychological stress: A metaanalysis. *Palliative & Supportive Care, 16*(5), 608–632.

Walker, J., Hansen, C. H., Martin, P., Symeonides, S., Gourley, C., Wall, L., Weller, D., Murray, G., Sharpe, M. , & SMaRT (Symptom Management Research Trials) Oncology-3 Team. (2014). Integrated collaborative care for major depression comorbid with a poor prognosis cancer (SMaRT Oncology-3): A multicentre randomised controlled trial in patients with lung cancer. *The Lancet Oncology, 15*(10), 1168–1176.

Watson, G. A., Saunders, J., & Coate, L. (2018). Evaluating the time to palliative care referrals in patients with small-cell lung cancer: A single-centre retrospective review. *American Journal of Hospice and Palliative Medicine, 35*(11), 1426–1432.

Wise, M., Marchand, L. R., Roberts, L. J., & Chih, M. Y. (2018). Suffering in advanced cancer: A randomized control trial of a narrative intervention. *Journal of Palliative Medicine, 21*(2), 200–207.

World Health Orgaization (WHO) Expert Committee on Cancer Pain Relief and Active Supportive Care & World Health Organization. (1990). Cancer pain relief and palliative care : Report of a WHO expert committee [meeting held in Geneva from 3 to 10 July 1989]. World Health Organization. https://apps.who.int/iris/handle/10665/39524

Zebrack, B., Kayser, K., Bybee, D., Padgett, L., Sundstrom, L., Jobin, C., & Oktay, J. (2017). A practice-based evaluation of distress screening protocol adherence and medical service utilization. *Journal of the National Comprehensive Cancer Network, 15*(7), 903–912.

Zebrack, B., Kayser, K., Sundstrom, L., Savas, S. A., Henrickson, C., Acquati, C., & Tamas, R. L. (2015). Psychosocial distress screening implementation in cancer care: An analysis of adherence, responsiveness, and acceptability. *Journal of Clinical Oncology, 33*(10), 1165–1170.

Zimmermann, C., Swami, N., Krzyzanowska, M., Hannon, B., Leighl, N., Oza, A., Moore, M., Rydall, A., Rodin, G., Tannock, I., Donner, A., & Lo, C. (2014). Early palliative care for patients with advanced cancer: A cluster-randomised controlled trial. *The Lancet, 383*(9930), 1721–1730.

Zimmermann, C., Yuen, D., Mischitelle, A., Minden, M. D., Brandwein, J. M., Schimmer, A., Gagliese, L., Lo, C., Rydall, A., & Rodin, G. (2013). Symptom burden and supportive care in patients with acute leukemia. *Leukemia Research, 37*(7), 731–736.

Zimmermann, F. F., Burrell, B., & Jordan, J. (2018). The acceptability and potential benefits of mindfulness-based interventions in improving psychological well-being for adults with advanced cancer: A systematic review. *Complementary Therapies in Clinical Practice, 30*, 68–78.

CHAPTER 10

Measuring Process and Outcome in CALM

INTRODUCTION

It was clear to us from the very beginning that Managing Cancer and Living Meaningfully (CALM) must be grounded in scientific evidence. We knew that rigorous demonstrations of its effectiveness would be required for CALM to be accepted in the world of medicine and implemented routinely as part of cancer care. We therefore ensured that the clinical and research programs of CALM were integrated from their conception. We designed phase I and phase II trials to determine the feasibility and preliminary impact of CALM on patients with advanced cancer and their families, and invested considerable effort in creating, modifying, and validating measures that would be relevant for patients with advanced disease and applicable to CALM therapy. In this chapter, we will describe the role of these measures in building the scientific evidence base for CALM and in informing CALM clinical practice.

MEASURING THE IMPACT OF CALM

Early qualitative studies of the impact of CALM on patients with advanced cancer provided strong initial evidence for its effectiveness. Led by Rinat Nissim, a psychologist and qualitative researcher on our CALM team, this research gave voice to patients facing life-threatening illness and generated powerful narratives that supported the benefit of CALM and the relevance of its four domains (see Chapter 15 of this volume). In free narratives and semi-structured interviews conducted by members of our research team, patients indicated that CALM positively and uniquely contributed to their cancer experience (Nissim et al., 2012). Specifically, patients reported that CALM provided them with the time and space to reflect and with a safe space to talk about sensitive issues such as death and dying. CALM also helped them navigate a complicated healthcare system, better understand and manage their relationships with others, and reduce the strain that cancer put on their relationships (Nissim et al., 2012). In CALM, patients felt treated as a "whole person" within the healthcare system, a benefit that was experienced as unique and profound in cancer care. Patients emphasized the importance of the empathic presence of the therapist, whom they perceived as a knowledgeable insider in the cancer system, in achieving these benefits. These early qualitative results reassured us that CALM provided the kind of experience for patients that we had intended. However, we recognized that quantitative evidence, regarded as the "gold standard" in medicine, would be the metric by which the effectiveness of CALM would be judged in the scientific community.

Generating quantitative evidence to demonstrate the effectiveness of a psychotherapeutic intervention is an enormous challenge in any circumstance, but is particularly difficult in the context of advanced disease. A successful clinical trial in this population must demonstrate benefit in psychological well-being in individuals who are facing a multitude of challenges related to the progression of disease and the growing burden of physical symptoms and functional disability. Moreover, even the most rigorous process of randomization in a controlled trial may not ensure similarity between the treatment and control groups on all relevant variables. Demonstrating a positive effect is even more difficult when patients who are not experiencing psychological distress at baseline are included in the trial. Nonetheless, we deemed it important to include these individuals to determine whether CALM could prevent distress, in addition to relieving it. Although including patients without significant distress at baseline made it more challenging to demonstrate the impact of CALM in lessening distress, our broad inclusion criteria helped shed light on who was most likely to benefit from the CALM intervention.

Perhaps our most important challenge in developing the CALM clinical trials was the relative paucity of appropriate measurement tools that had been validated in an advanced cancer population for constructs relevant to CALM. Although scales had been developed for constructs such as death anxiety, attachment security, and quality of life, most had been validated in healthy or nonclinical populations or with patients who were not suffering from advanced disease. Their relevance in the context of an advanced and life-threatening illness was therefore not clear. As a result, much of our early work involved modifying and developing appropriate scales that would serve to assess CALM outcomes. For instance, many measures of death anxiety, an important target of CALM, had been validated mainly in nonclinical populations. These measures were often lengthy (Lester, 1994; Wittkowski, 2001) and included items that may not be relevant for patients with advanced disease (Triplett et al., 1995; Wong et al., 1994) or that limited the ability to detect change owing to intervention (e.g., Conte et al., 1982). Led by Chris Lo, we therefore developed the Death and Dying Distress Scale (DADDS), a brief, 15-item measure assessing distress related to death and dying (see Appendix A). This tool was validated with data obtained from patients with advanced disease (Lo, Hales, et al., 2011; Shapiro et al., 2020) and has become an important component of our CALM clinical and research programs.

Measures of attachment security, which plays an important role in CALM therapy (see Chapter 4 of this volume), had also not been adapted for individuals who may be older, in long-term stable romantic relationships, and suffering from advanced or life-threatening illness. To that end, our team modified and shortened an existing scale of adult attachment, the Experience in Close Relationships Scale (ECR; Brennan et al., 1998), to create a measure that would be relevant for an older population of patients for whom there may be many attachment figures, including their healthcare providers. The revised 16-item ECR-M16 was validated with patients with advanced disease (Lo et al., 2009; see Appendix B). Although we did not expect attachment security, which is a relatively stable personality characteristic, to be modified by CALM, the ECR-M16 has proved to be an extremely valuable tool both clinically and in our research. In our clinical work, it has allowed us to understand and quantify the difficulty patients may experience in relying upon others, in finding relief of distress through their attachment relationships, and in tolerating the dependency that is inevitably imposed by advanced disease. In our research, it has allowed us to demonstrate the effects of a secure attachment orientation in protecting against depression and other manifestations of distress (Rodin et al., 2007).

Finally, to ensure we had a reliable, appropriate measure of quality of life for advanced cancer patients, we examined the psychometric properties of the Quality of Life at the End of Life scale (QUAL-E; Steinhauser et al., 2002), which was originally developed based on qualitative research of perceptions of a good death (Steinhauser et al., 2000). We developed a shortened version of the QUAL-E tailored specifically to individuals with advanced cancer, named the Quality of Life at the End of Life-Cancer Scale

(QUAL-EC), which was first validated for research in early palliative care (Lo, Burman, et al., 2011; see Appendix C). The availability of this brief, validated scale of quality of life for patients with advanced cancer has allowed us to assess relevant CALM outcomes such as patients' perceived relationship with healthcare providers, preparation for the end of life, and life completion.

SELECTING APPROPRIATE OUTCOME MEASURES

Choosing appropriate outcome measures for a randomized controlled trial (RCT) of a psychotherapeutic intervention for patients with advanced disease is essential, but it presents risks. Different outcomes may be relevant for different patients, but traditional RCTs do not allow for individual tailoring of outcomes. Within these constraints, we selected depression, as measured by the Patient Health Questionnaire-9 (PHQ-9; Kroenke et al., 2001; see Appendix D), as the primary outcome of the CALM RCT because we had the most evidence for the high prevalence of depression in advanced cancer (e.g., Lo et al., 2010; Mitchell et al., 2011), for its association with the multiple challenges of advanced disease (e.g., Fitzgerald et al., 2015; Lo et al., 2010), and for its responsiveness to therapeutic interventions (e.g., Li et al., 2012). Our earlier work identified depression as a final common pathway of distress in patients with advanced cancer (Rodin et al., 2009), and we hypothesized that the benefit of CALM would be achieved through its effect on a variety of factors along this pathway. Although multiple secondary outcomes were included, such as posttraumatic growth, demoralization, and spiritual well-being, we postulated that death anxiety (measured by the DADDS) and quality of life at the end of life (measured by the QUAL-EC) were the most likely of these to be influenced by CALM therapy, due to the nature of CALM and its domains (see Chapter 15 of this volume).

The results of our large CALM RCT demonstrated that patients treated with CALM showed greater improvement of depressive symptoms at three months than did patients who received usual care alone, and an even greater effect at six months (Rodin et al., 2018). Among patients who were not depressed at baseline, those who received CALM were less likely to be depressed at three months than were patients receiving usual care, indicating that CALM may have a preventive effect on depressive symptoms. This finding suggests, in turn, that CALM may improve resilience and adaptation during the course of advanced cancer. Patients who received CALM also reported better death preparation and less death anxiety, implying that CALM may enhance the capacity for advance care planning. The latter benefits were particularly evident in patients with moderate levels of death anxiety at the start of the treatment.

BEYOND OUTCOME MEASURES

By demonstrating effects on primary and secondary outcome measures, the CALM RCT provided compelling evidence for the benefit of CALM. However, like many other psychotherapeutic interventions, the "magic ingredient" of CALM that accounts for its effectiveness is more difficult to demonstrate. Measures assessing the process and integrity of an intervention—that is, of whether it is delivered as it was intended—have been developed to open this "black box" and determine how psychotherapeutic interventions work. Building on the work of David Spiegel and James Spira (1991), we developed a CALM Treatment Integrity Measure (CTIM; Rodin et al., 2018) to assess the extent to which CALM is delivered in accordance with its basic tenets (see Appendix E). Based on case presentations by therapists and review of recorded sessions, the CTIM allows for a rating of elements of the therapeutic process. These include the empathic understanding and responsiveness of the therapist; the extent to which reflective awareness is supported, professional boundaries are maintained, and the therapist is engaged with the patient; the extent to which the therapist is able to help the patient modulate affect, think about, and manage negative events and emotions; adjust the frame between supportive exploratory and problem-solving approaches; and attend to the content and timing of the sessions, as needed. This process-focused measure also assesses the extent to which all four domains of CALM are addressed.

Because the CTIM is an objective observer-rated measure of treatment integrity, it does not necessarily capture the experience of the patient. To that end, our team developed a measure to assess the extent to which patients perceive benefit from the process and content of CALM. The Clinical Evaluation Questionnaire (CEQ) is a 7-item questionnaire in which items are rated by patients on a 5-point scale (Lo et al., 2015; de Vries et al., 2020; see Appendix F). It was administered to all participants in the CALM RCT at the three- and six-month endpoints, allowing them to rate the extent to which CALM provided them with a reflective space, allowed them to better express and manage their feelings, and addressed concerns in each of the four CALM domains. Based on preliminary factor analyses, the CEQ has a high internal consistency and appears to capture one underlying construct (de Vries et al., 2020).

The CEQ can be regarded as both a process and outcome measure of CALM. Process in healthcare has been defined as the method by which healthcare is provided (Donabedian, 1980). This is distinguished from structure, which is the environment in which healthcare is provided, and from outcome, which is the consequence of healthcare. The findings of the CEQ can be considered to assess both process and outcome in CALM in that they reflect the extent to which a patient experiences benefit from the specific dimensions of the CALM process. While more attention tends to be paid to measures of outcomes than to process, particularly in RCTs, the process of the intervention in psychotherapy may be as important to the patient as the quantitative outcomes. Process measures may better capture the benefit of the intervention as perceived by the patient, and be less likely than outcome measures to be affected by the many other factors that affect the quality of care (Lilford et al., 2007). Indeed, depression in patients with advanced disease receiving CALM is typically affected by such factors as the progression or recurrence of disease, the physical symptom burden, or the receipt of negative test results.

Patients receiving CALM in our RCT reported higher total CEQ scores than the usual care group (de Vries et al., 2020). Moreover, patients receiving CALM rated six of the seven individual items on the CEQ more highly than did individuals who were receiving usual care alone. The item on which these groups did not differ enquired about the benefit of freely discussing concerns about their cancer and treatment options. The lack of difference on this item between those receiving CALM and those receiving usual care may not be surprising, since discussions about cancer and its treatment are the primary focus of cancer clinic interactions. Nonetheless, these CEQ results highlight the perceived benefits of CALM and indicate that the intervention was providing patients with what was intended. A positive relationship between number of CALM sessions and CEQ scores further suggests an additive benefit from CALM sessions (de Vries et al., 2020).

Of note, patients' CEQ scores at three and six months did not correlate with their scores on many of the primary and secondary outcome measures at these time points, including on measures of depression and death anxiety (de Vries et al., 2020). Scores on the CEQ did correlate with two subscales of the QUAL-EC (relationship with healthcare providers and life completion), and, in those receiving CALM, with spiritual well-being. These findings suggest that the perceived benefit of the therapy for patients is linked to meaningful and practical outcomes near the end of life. However, the lack of association of the CEQ with our primary and secondary distress outcomes deserves consideration.

The disconnection between CEQ scores and the outcomes of depression and death anxiety may be because different mechanisms drive the effect of CALM on depression and death anxiety compared to the CEQ. Whereas measures of depression and death anxiety reflect symptoms of distress, the CEQ captures the experience of therapy and its perceived impact on unique and perhaps more personal outcomes, such as self-understanding. As one participant in the RCT reported, "Coping with cancer is an ongoing process with ups and downs, and new issues that come to light, and the session helps me understand and frame my understanding." It is also possible that the CEQ allows for a more uniformly positive effect of CALM to be demonstrated, whereas symptoms of depression and death anxiety may be influenced by many factors unrelated to CALM, such as disease progression or pain. Thus, an intermediate process measure such as the CEQ may not be linked to quantitative outcomes due to a low signal-to-noise ratio resulting from the occurrence of intervening variables in the course of advanced disease.

THE INTEGRATION OF RESEARCH MEASURES INTO CLINICAL CARE

We have found that the administration of quantitative measures at the onset of CALM and at subsequent time points is useful not only to assess outcomes but also to enhance the integrity and quality of the intervention. Scores on these measures can support the therapist in the approach that is being taken or point to difficulties that have not yet been adequately addressed. At the least, the lack of concordance between measurement scores and the experience of the therapist can be examined. Some patients feel more comfortable reporting difficulties on a self-report questionnaire than they do raising these issues directly with their therapist. Elevated scores on these measures may reflect a patient's first step in introducing their distress into the therapy. In other cases, unexpectedly high scores may reflect the avoidance or reluctance of the therapist to address a sensitive or difficult area and can alert therapists to its importance for the patient. Further, the results on test scores may help therapists to conceptualize and formulate the difficulties of their patients and to guide specific therapeutic interventions. In particular, the ECR-M16, the DADDS, and the CEQ are regularly used to improve the CALM therapy process.

Although we did not expect attachment security to be modified by CALM, the ECR-M16 has nonetheless been an extremely valuable tool.

It has allowed therapists to confirm their clinical impression of the patient's attachment security, has guided attachment-related therapeutic interventions, and has allowed for the assessment of changes in this domain. The ECR-M16 generates scores on avoidant and anxious attachment styles (Lo et al., 2009), which can help explain problematic relationships and interactions with close others or healthcare providers and can shed light on the fears and wishes of the patient in the relationship with the therapist (Tan et al., 2005). Those with high attachment avoidance tend to underreport distress and dismiss the need to rely on others, including the therapist. It may take more time for such patients to develop a meaningful relationship with the therapist that can serve to modulate their distress. Such individuals may benefit from approaches that support their autonomy and confirm their strengths and capacities. Those who are more anxiously attached tend to be fearful that sufficient support will not be available and their distress may easily escalate (see Chapter 4 of this volume). These patients may benefit most from predictability and reliability in the therapeutic relationship.

Although high levels of death anxiety are reported by almost half of patients with metastatic cancer (Eggen et al., 2020), and open-ended questions can elicit these concerns, even in the first CALM session (Shaw et al., 2017), death-related anxieties can often be avoided by both patients and therapists. High scores on the DADDS may indicate that a supportive intervention is required to lower levels of distress before reflection can occur. Patients with moderate levels of death anxiety that are within a window of tolerance may be better able to reflect on such concerns (Tong et al., 2016). We found that such patients were most likely to have a significant reduction in death anxiety as a result of participating in CALM (Rodin et al., 2018). Patients with very low scores may report little distress about dying and death because they have come to accept the end of life, or because they are unwilling or unable to reflect on such concerns. The latter may be more feasible to maintain when there is a lack of physical symptoms or of visible manifestations of the disease and may reflect an avoidant attachment style.

Finally, the CEQ can be used to directly evaluate the CALM therapy process. Lower scores on any of the items of the CEQ after three months can indicate a need to adjust the therapeutic intervention accordingly. This feedback loop can be powerful in improving therapeutic effectiveness with a particular patient. CEQ scores at three months and at the end of therapy can help therapists learn from each case and improve and refine their therapeutic skills.

CONCLUSION

Mixed-methods research with both qualitative and quantitative components may be the most informative approach to understanding the impact of an intervention. Our qualitative research has been particularly valuable in understanding the experience of advanced disease and of CALM. The quantitative measures that we have modified and validated for patients with advanced disease have been essential in ensuring the integrity of the CALM intervention and in demonstrating its ability to improve depression, death anxiety, and preparation for the end of life. The CEQ has provided additional intermediate evidence of the benefit of CALM in relation to its domains from the perspective of the patient. However, further research is needed to understand the lack of relationship between scores on the CEQ and on quantitative measures of distress. The availability of relevant, validated quantitative measures for depression, death anxiety, attachment, quality of life, and the patient's perspective of the CALM process has proven to be extremely valuable for the delivery of CALM. Patient's scores on these measures can serve to guide therapists in the regulation of affect, the nature of support that is needed, and the content domains that require attention. The PHQ-9, DADDS, ECR-M16, and the CEQ are therefore now routinely integrated into CALM treatment.

REFERENCES

Brennan, K. A., Clark, C. L., & Shaver, P. R. (1998). Self-report measurement of adult attachment: An integrative overview. In J. A. Simpson & W. S. Rholes (Eds.), *Attachment theory and close relationships* (pp. 46–76). Guilford Press.

Conte, H. R., Weiner, M. B., & Plutchik, R. (1982). Measuring death anxiety: Conceptual, psychometric, and factor-analytic aspects. *Journal of Personality and Social Psychology, 43*(4), 775–785.

de Vries, F. E., Mah, K., Shapiro, G. K., Rydall, A., Hales, S., & Rodin, G. (2020). Assessing the process of a brief psychotherapy for patients with advanced cancer. (Submitted for publication).

Donabedian, A. (1980). *Explorations in quality assessment and monitoring: The definition of quality and approaches to its assessment* (Vol. 1). Health Administration Press.

Eggen, A. C., Reyners, A. K. L., Shen, G., Bosma, I., Jalving, M., Leighl, N. B., Liu, G., Richard, N. M., Mah, K., Schultz, D. B., Edelstein, K., & Rodin, G. (2020). Death anxiety in patients with metastatic non-small cell lung cancer with and without brain metastases. *Journal of Pain and Symptom Management, 60*(2), 422–429.

Fitzgerald, P., Lo, C., Li, M., Gagliese, L., Zimmermann, C., & Rodin, G. (2015). The relationship between depression and physical symptom burden in advanced cancer. *BMJ Supportive & Palliative Care, 5*(4), 381–388.

Kroenke, K., Spitzer, R. L., & Williams, J. B. (2001). The PHQ-9: Validity of a brief depression severity measure. *Journal of General Internal Medicine, 16*(9), 606–613.

Lester, D. (1994). The Collett–Lester Fear of Death Scale. In R. A. Neimeyer (Ed.), *Series in death education, aging, and health care. Death anxiety handbook: Research, instrumentation, and application* (pp. 45–60). Taylor & Francis.

Li, M., Fitzgerald, P., & Rodin, G. (2012). Evidence-based treatment of depression in patients with cancer. *Journal of Clinical Oncology, 30*(11), 1187–1196.

Lilford, R. J., Brown, C. A., & Nicholl, J. (2007). Use of process measures to monitor the quality of clinical practice. *BMJ, 335*(7621), 648–650.

Lo, C., Burman, D., Swami, N., Gagliese, L., Rodin, G., & Zimmermann, C. (2011). Validation of the QUAL-EC for assessing quality of life in patients with advanced cancer. *European Journal of Cancer, 47*(4), 554–560.

Lo, C., Hales, S., Rydall, A., Panday, T., Chiu, A., Malfitano, C., Jung, J., Li, M., Nissim, R., Zimmermann, C., & Rodin, G. (2015). Managing Cancer And Living Meaningfully: Study protocol for a randomized controlled trial. *Trials, 16*, 391. doi: 10.1186/s13063-015-0811-1.

Lo, C., Hales, S., Zimmermann, C., Gagliese, L., Rydall, A., & Rodin, G. (2011). Measuring death-related anxiety in advanced cancer: Preliminary psychometrics of the Death and Dying Distress Scale. *Journal of Pediatric Hematology/Oncology, 33*(Suppl 2), S140–S145.

Lo, C., Walsh, A., Mikulincer, M., Gagliese, L., Zimmermann, C., & Rodin, G. (2009). Measuring attachment security in patients with advanced cancer: Psychometric properties of a modified and brief Experiences in Close Relationships scale. *Psycho-Oncology, 18*(5), 490–499.

Lo, C., Zimmermann, C., Rydall, A., Walsh, A., Jones, J. M., Moore, M. J., Shepherd, F. A., Gagliese, L., & Rodin, G. (2010). Longitudinal study of depressive symptoms in patients with metastatic gastrointestinal and lung cancer. *Journal of Clinical Oncology, 28*(18), 3084–3089.

Mitchell, A. J., Chan, M., Bhatti, H., Halton, M., Grassi, L., Johansen, C., & Meader, N. (2011). Prevalence of depression, anxiety, and adjustment disorder in oncological, haematological, and palliative-care settings: A meta-analysis of 94 interview-based studies. *The Lancet Oncology, 12*(2), 160–174.

Nissim, R., Freeman, E., Lo, C., Zimmermann, C., Gagliese, L., Rydall, A., Hales, S., & Rodin, G. (2012). Managing Cancer and Living Meaningfully (CALM): A qualitative study of a brief individual psychotherapy for individuals with advanced cancer. *Palliative Medicine, 26*(5), 713–721.

Rodin, G., Lo, C., Mikulincer, M., Donner, A., Gagliese, L., & Zimmermann, C. (2009). Pathways to distress: The multiple determinants of depression, hopelessness, and the desire for hastened death in metastatic cancer patients. *Social Science & Medicine, 68*(3), 562–569.

Rodin, G., Lo, C., Rydall, A., Shnall, J. Malfinato, C., Chiu, A., Panday, T., Watt, S., An, E., Nissim, R., Li, M., Zimmermann, C., & Hales, S. (2018). Managing Cancer and Living Meaningfully (CALM): A randomized controlled trial of a psychological intervention for patients with advanced cancer. *Journal of Clinical Oncology, 36*(23), 2422–2432.

Rodin, G., Walsh, A., Zimmermann, C., Gagliese, L., Jones, J., Shepherd, F. A., Moore, M., Braun, M., Donner, A., & Mikulincer, M. (2007). The contribution of attachment security and social support to depressive symptoms in patients with metastatic cancer. *Psycho-Oncology, 16*(12), 1080–1091.

Shapiro, G. K., Mah, K., Li, M., Zimmermann, C., Hales, S., & Rodin, G. (2020). Validation of the Death and Dying Distress Scale in patients with advanced cancer. *Psycho-Oncology.* 2020 Dec 26. doi: 10.1002/pon.5620. Epub ahead of print.

Shaw, C., Chrysikou, V., Davis, S., Gessler, S., Rodin, G., & Lanceley, A. (2017). Inviting end-of-life talk in initial CALM therapy sessions: A conversation analytic study. *Patient Education and Counseling, 100*(2), 259–266.

Spiegel, D., & Spira, J. (1991). *Supportive-expressive group therapy: A treatment manual of psychosocial intervention for women with metastatic breast cancer.* Stanford University School of Medicine.

Steinhauser, K. E., Bosworth, H. B., Clipp, E. C., McNeilly, M., Christakis, N. A., Parker, J., & Tulsky, J. A. (2002). Initial assessment of a new instrument to measure quality of life at the end of life. *Journal of Palliative Medicine, 5*(6), 829–841.

Steinhauser, K. E., Christakis, N. A., Clipp, E. C., McNeilly, M., McIntyre, L., & Tulsky, J. A. (2000). Factors considered important at the end of life by patients, family, physicians, and other care providers. *JAMA, 284*(19), 2476–2482.

Tan, A., Zimmermann, C., & Rodin, G. (2005). Interpersonal processes in palliative care: An attachment perspective on the patient-clinician relationship. *Palliative Medicine, 19*(2), 143–150.

Tong, E., Deckert, A., Gani, N., Nissim, R., Rydall, A., Hales, S., Rodin, G., & Lo, C. (2016). The meaning of self-reported death anxiety in advanced cancer. *Palliative Medicine, 30*(8), 772–779.

Triplett, G., Cohen, D., Reimer, W., Rinaldi, S., Hill, C., Roshdieh, S., Stanczak, E. M., Siscoe, K., & Templer, D. I. (1995). Death discomfort differential. *OMEGA— Journal of Death and Dying, 31*(4), 295–304.

Wittkowski, J. (2001). The construction of the Multidimensional Orientation Toward Dying and Death Inventory (MODDI-F). *Death Studies, 25*(6), 479–495.

Wong, P. T. P., Reker, G. T., & Gesser, G. R. A. (1994). Death Attitude Profile– Revised: A multidimensional measure of attitudes toward death. In R. A. Neimeyer (Ed.), *Series in death education, aging, and health care. Death handbook: Research, instrumentation, and application* (pp. 121–148). Taylor & Francis.

CHAPTER 11

The Experience of CALM Training

It's just a hugely positive experience being exposed and part of the group, really. I feel part of a wider CALM community.

—CALM workshop participant

INTRODUCTION

Early in the process of developing Managing Cancer and Living Meaningfully (CALM), we began to engage in teaching and supervision activities locally, nationally, and internationally. This engagement created a valuable iterative process whereby feedback, criticism, experience, and ideas from our colleagues furthered our thinking and aided in the improvement and development of CALM. These activities also helped build a mutually supportive community of clinicians and researchers from around the globe engaged in CALM. Our colleagues from different countries shared with us their struggles to meet the psychological needs of patients facing advanced disease and noted the lack of an evidence-based framework for their work. Those with a psychotherapeutic background had been providing psychological care that naturally included elements of CALM but they were looking for a more explicit framework and structure for teaching and research. CALM answered this need.

Many clinicians reported that CALM offered support and validation for their work in cancer centers, where there was often greater focus on cancer and anticancer treatment than on the persons affected by the illness and where trainees and staff did not feel adequately prepared to support patients and families living with advanced disease. The CALM workshops, case supervision, and advanced training have created a valuable community of practice and support for our colleagues, which has helped them advocate within their settings for CALM to become a standard of care. The words of some of our colleagues and collaborators, included in the epilogue of this book, give some indication of what CALM has meant to them in their settings in different parts of the world.

THE BENEFIT OF CALM AND CALM TRAINING FOR CLINICIANS

CALM training provides a framework for therapists to respond to the distress of patients with advanced cancer and their families. It also offers a parallel experience of support for clinicians, in which they are provided the reflective space to consider their own feelings about living in the face of mortality. As part of our CALM training program, we have been invested in teaching, not only to ensure the integrity and quality of the intervention for patients and families, but also to provide clinicians with more generalizable knowledge and skills to support them in their care of patients living with advanced and life-threatening disease. The psychotherapy education literature suggests that the most effective training programs for mental health professionals involve a combination of didactic teaching, supervised case evaluation, ongoing advanced training, and the assessment of patient outcomes (Fairburn & Cooper, 2011; Herschell et al., 2010). We have been careful to attend to these elements when designing our training program, which includes a continuum of (a) introductory workshops that incorporate didactic teaching, case-based application of the CALM framework, and experiential learning; (b) clinical case supervision offered via group supervision meetings; and (c) ongoing advanced workshops for practicing clinicians focused on more advanced topics.

Psychotherapy training is always challenging, given the complex nature of psychotherapeutic interventions and the importance of nonverbal and less structured elements in psychotherapeutic care. Preserving the complexity and flexibility of an intervention while also breaking it down into teachable components is complicated in any situation, but is heightened in CALM training due to the diverse settings and cultures in which it is delivered and the wide range of disciplines and prior theoretical frameworks of its trainees. Nonetheless, we have successfully trained a wide variety of care providers in CALM therapy, including oncologists, palliative care physicians, psychiatrists, psychologists, nurses, social workers, spiritual care providers, and occupational therapists. Our success in doing so may be related to the fact that all of these professionals had already been involved in meaningful conversations of one kind or another with patients with advanced disease and their families.

All clinicians trained in CALM receive instruction in its basic principles, and each brings to the intervention their own unique knowledge and expertise from their clinical background. More advanced training has been developed for clinicians who have had prior CALM training and are using it in their practice. In both our introductory and advanced workshops, we use real cases to illustrate how CALM is applied both in the moment and over the course of therapy. Case summaries, live examples of clinical encounters with actors, and videos of actual CALM sessions have been presented during CALM training, with the latter tending to be the most engaging for clinicians. Witnessing actual CALM therapists interview patients with advanced disease and then practicing CALM skills with trained actors and reflecting on these experiences has been reported by trainees as the most valuable aspect of training. By showing real therapist–patient interactions, we have been able to shed light on what CALM therapists actually do in a way that words cannot easily convey.

Introductory workshops serve as both an orientation to the CALM approach and a foundation for further training. Many clinicians find that these workshops provide them with tools that can be applied to a wide range of clinical encounters. Some choose to pursue CALM training in more depth through ongoing case supervision and to become certified as CALM therapists. Some may even progress further to become certified as CALM supervisors. CALM supervision takes place in person and online, usually in a group format. The group format is not only efficient but also provides clinicians with a highly valuable shared experience and collegial support for the complex problems and intense feelings that may emerge during the process of therapy.

As part of our training program of workshops and supervision, we have conducted both quantitative and qualitative evaluations. Trainees report a high level of satisfaction with the CALM workshops, with almost all indicating that the principles of CALM could be applied to their clinical work. Most clinicians also report an intention to pursue further training. Based on standardized questionnaires, we found a significant increase in self-reported empathy among attendees following the workshop, an effect that was greatest among those without previous psychotherapy training. Qualitative post-workshop interviews supported these findings, with clinicians new to the psychosocial care of patients with advanced disease or to psychotherapeutic care in general finding workshops and training opportunities most beneficial. More experienced clinicians stated that they appreciated CALM's explicit framework and evidence base, which allowed them to advocate for funding and resources within their institutions. They also frequently remarked on the potential value of the CALM approach for teaching trainees within their sites and disciplines.

Workshop attendees consistently reported feeling inspired and supported in their clinical work, which they often felt was undervalued and unsupported in their profession or institution. Joining the CALM community provided a sense of belonging, encouragement for their work, and a space in which to reflect. As one participant noted, "I found that it actually profoundly influenced what I was doing in terms of my thinking . . . I was so mindful after the course, of how . . . to actually allow space for this process to unfold." Another talked about feeling like a "lone ranger" in her small center and that CALM training provided a sense of connection with other practitioners that was encouraging and sustaining. We have found similar themes of the benefits of the group, support, and space to reflect in qualitative research evaluating the experience of our peer supervision groups.

The ongoing development of the CALM training workshops and supervision has helped establish an international community of CALM practice. Such communities, which exist across a range of disciplines and activities, can become models of collective learning that build skills and relationships that support knowledge creation and professional identity formation (Li et al., 2009; Wenger, 1998). This has been the case with CALM training, which has not only ensured the integrity of the intervention but has also fostered collegial support and provided attendees with an opportunity to reflect. Many have gone on to implement CALM training and program development in their own settings. There have been remarkable examples of this occurring in various settings ranging from China and Japan to Europe, and North and South America. Leaders in these sites have become experts in CALM delivery and now work with our Global CALM program (see Chapter 12 of this volume) to build strong networks of CALM practice in their countries.

CONCLUSION

We have found that the process of CALM training, through workshops and case supervision, has been essential to ensure the integrity and consistency of CALM as delivered by different clinicians across different settings. It has also fostered advancement of the intervention, therapist skill development, collegial support, and an opportunity for reflection, and has helped therapists to develop realistic but meaningful expectations in the face of impending mortality. CALM workshops and training have been a valuable education pathway for attendees, many of whom go on to become certified in CALM and lead implementation in their own settings.

REFERENCES

Fairburn, C. G., & Cooper, Z. (2011). Therapist competence, therapy quality, and therapist training. *Behaviour Research and Therapy, 49*(6-7), 373–378.

Herschell, A. D., Kolko, D. J., Baumann, B. L., & Davis, A. C. (2010). The role of therapist training in the implementation of psychosocial treatments: A review and critique with recommendations. *Clinical Psychology Review, 30*(4), 448–466.

Li, L. C., Grimshaw, J. M., Nielsen, C., Judd, M., Coyte, P. C., & Graham, I. D. (2009). Evolution of Wenger's concept of community of practice. *Implementation Science, 4*, 11. doi: 10.1186/1748-5908-4-11.

Wenger, E. (1998). Communities of practice: Learning as a social system. *Systems Thinker, 9*(5), 2–3.

CHAPTER 12

From Our Clinic, Across the Globe

CALM Training, Research, and Advocacy

Our patients are distressed. Our patients need help. We finally have a resource available in CALM.

—Ashlee Loughlan, Site Lead (Virginia)

Just as Laozi said in the Tao Te Ching, "The Tao never strives, yet nothing is left undone." That is what CALM therapy is.

—Yeong-Yuh Juang, Site Lead (Taiwan)

INTRODUCTION

Managing Cancer and Living Meaningfully (CALM) grew out of our clinical and research work at the Princess Margaret Cancer Centre in Toronto, Canada, one of the most multicultural cities in the world. More than half of the population of this city belong to a visible minority group, with more than 250 ethnic or cultural origins represented. It has the highest per capita immigration rate in the world with almost half of the population being immigrants to Canada (Statistics Canada, 2019a, 2019b). Living and working in this environment has kept issues of culture, language, and identity in the forefront of our minds, with the hope that CALM could be applied across a broad range of cultures and languages in our clinic, our city, and the world.

Over the last decade, the response to CALM from colleagues across the globe has been overwhelmingly positive. Clinicians have uniformly found CALM to be highly adaptable to their cultures, settings, and institutions.

Many have become partners in the dissemination of CALM, publishing and presenting findings from their settings, participating in international training workshops, and providing feedback that has helped to shape and strengthen the intervention. We have now trained thousands of clinicians across the globe, many returning year after year to attend our international advanced workshops. They have supported our view that CALM should be considered an essential and standard element of psychosocial care for patients with advanced cancer around the world and have joined us in advocating for this to become realized.

UNIVERSALITY AND ADAPTABILITY OF CALM

All psychotherapeutic approaches carry a risk of ethnocentricity because of inherent biases and assumptions that may not generalize across cultures (Tseng, 2001). However, the success of CALM across diverse settings and populations indicates that this may be less problematic in CALM than in other interventions. We believe that the generalizability of CALM across cultures may be the result of several important factors. Most importantly, the problems and fears that individuals with advanced disease face are universal, and the domains of CALM designed to address these fears are therefore relevant in all cultures and settings. Further, because CALM is a semi-structured rather than a prescriptive intervention, it can be delivered in the voice, language, and cultural idiom of the therapist. The contextual application of CALM in diverse cultural settings is supported by relational theory, which highlights that meaning is not imposed or discovered, but is developed in relationship with others (Aron & Lechich, 2012). From this perspective, the therapist's stance is one of being a nonexpert on the inner world of the patient, and the therapeutic project is one of co-investigation and co-discovery. CALM requires therapists to consider their own world views and orientations and to reflect on their interplay with those of the patient and their family.

Attention to the individual patient and to the family context is another aspect of CALM that has been welcomed across communities. Consistent with the philosophy of palliative care, advanced cancer is viewed in CALM as a family problem and a major goal of the intervention is to strengthen the support available from and for the family. For this reason, caregivers are routinely invited into the therapy for a single session and, in many cases, for the entire course of therapy.

An overarching aspect of CALM that has contributed to its vibrancy and spread is the spirit of inquiry that drives the work and its development. When we teach, we strive to learn from and to collaborate with our students and participants. We continue to examine how CALM can be applied in diverse settings, in which there may be great variation in the acceptability of or comfort with emotional communication; in the role that spouses, parents, and other family members play; in the concerns of patients related to dependency and family burden; and in attitudes about the end of life. We have aimed wherever we travel and present CALM to be curious and interested in the clinicians with whom we are working, and in their patients, clinics, and communities.

GLOBAL CALM: A PROGRAM OF TRAINING AND RESEARCH

In 2018, the Global Institute of Psychosocial, Palliative, and End-of-Life Care (GIPPEC; www.gippec.org) launched the Global CALM Training Program. A University of Toronto research institute dedicated to global research and clinical collaboration, GIPPEC was established to support interdisciplinary research, education, and advocacy related to advanced disease. GIPPEC, based at the Princess Margaret Cancer Centre, has supported the Global CALM program alongside Movember, a Melbourne, Australia–based international agency promoting clinical care and research to improve the well-being of those living with prostate and other cancers.

The Global CALM Training Program was designed to build capacity for CALM internationally, to educate healthcare providers in CALM through workshops and clinical supervision, and to advance global knowledge through research collaboration and international exchange. The program is a vehicle for structured training, clinical implementation, and research, and facilitates the routine implementation of psychosocial interventions of this kind in cancer. It works to overcome barriers to CALM implementation by investigating and addressing the cultural modifications that may be required across diverse regions and cultures. Clinicians, educators, and researchers from North and South America, Europe, the Middle East, Asia, and Australia are actively participating in the Global CALM implementation project, representing a global community with shared expertise and experience in the implementation and investigation of CALM. Research conducted by these colleagues has been presented at international meetings and published in peer reviewed journals (e.g., Caruso, Sabato, et al., 2020; Engelmann et al., 2016; Mehnert et al., 2020; Scheffold, Wollbruck et al., 2015; Scheffold et al., 2017; Troncoso et al., 2019).

There has been strong and dedicated leadership from international sites that have joined the Global CALM program. Since 2018, 18 global sites and 7 Canadian sites have actively participated in the Global CALM program, some of which have initiated their own CALM-related research studies in collaboration with the Global CALM team in Toronto, Canada (see Figure 12.1 for levels of CALM implementation).

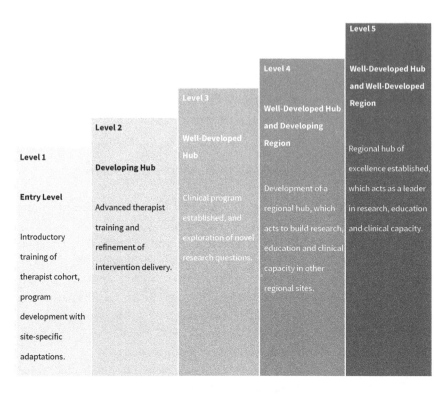

Figure 12.1. Levels of CALM implementation

The Global CALM Training Program has employed a train-the-trainer model. After attending a workshop, clinicians begin by seeing CALM patients in their centers and receive online international supervision involving case review, conceptualization, and discussion among clinicians from across the world. Upon certification as a CALM therapist, clinicians can then pursue training to become a CALM supervisor. The goal is for CALM supervisors and leads to sustain and expand CALM research and clinical practice in their region.

GLOBAL CALM RESEARCH

The spirit of inquiry has been intrinsic to the CALM project from its inception, and research and knowledge translation have been embedded within all of its activities. The first CALM manual, which documented the foundations and practice of this new intervention, was written for an initial pilot study (Rodin et al., Copyright 2015). Results of this pilot were promising, with participants describing five unique benefits of the intervention: a safe place to process the experience of advanced cancer, permission to talk about death and dying, assistance in managing the illness and navigating the healthcare system, resolution of relational strain, and an opportunity to "be seen as a whole person" within the healthcare system (Nissim et al., 2012, p. 716). These effects of CALM were experienced by participants as unique and not encountered elsewhere in their cancer care. The qualitative results were supported by a quantitative non-randomized pilot trial, which found that CALM was associated with a reduction in depressive symptoms and death anxiety and an increase in spiritual well-being at three and six months after therapy initiation (Lo et al., 2014). A subsequent randomized feasibility pilot trial demonstrated the feasibility of delivering CALM to patients with advanced disease, and provided further support for potential treatment effects on depression symptoms, attachment anxiety and attachment avoidance (Lo et al., 2019).

The next step in our research program was to conduct a phase III randomized controlled trial, which recruited more than 300 patients with metastatic cancer from oncology clinics at our center and compared CALM to usual care (Rodin et al., 2018). The primary outcome for this study was the severity of depressive symptoms and secondary outcomes included distress related to death and dying, attachment security, spiritual well-being, quality of life, posttraumatic growth, and satisfaction with care. This study found significantly greater improvements in depressive symptoms and end-of-life preparation in the CALM treatment arm compared to usual care. It also found that patients who were not depressed at baseline were less likely to become depressed at the three- and six-month follow-ups, suggesting a preventive effect. Those with moderate levels of distress about dying and death benefited most from CALM therapy in terms of reduction of such distress and improvement in generalized anxiety, demoralization, spiritual well-being, and attachment security. Participants receiving CALM also reported significantly greater benefit on all CALM-specific dimensions of well-being than did those receiving usual care based on their ratings on the Clinical Evaluation Questionnaire (de Vries et al., 2020; see Chapter 10 of this volume).

An expanding international program of research has emerged following our initial studies, with support from our Global CALM program. This program has promoted CALM research within diverse settings, cultures, and languages. Research trials in Germany (Koranyi et al., 2020; Mehnert et al., 2020; Scheffold, Philipp, et al., 2015; Scheffold, Wollbruck, et al., 2015) and Italy (Caruso, Nanni, et al., 2020; Caruso, Sabato, et al., 2020) have been completed with promising results. Pilot studies are now underway in other sites within North America, Europe, and Asia, demonstrating the relevance and applicability of CALM in diverse settings. To achieve more universal access to CALM for those unable to access in-person therapy, an internet-based psychoeducational intervention called iCALM is now in development jointly with colleagues in Ulm, Germany.

CONCLUSION

The fears and hopes of individuals with advanced disease and their families are remarkably similar across the world, despite variations in culture, language, religion, family structure, nature of government, resources, and healthcare systems. CALM addresses these hopes and fears, and the shared problems of these individuals with flexibility and adaptability to accommodate individual and cultural differences. The Global CALM project was established to train clinicians of multiple disciplines in the delivery of the intervention and to attract resources and support for CALM to become a global standard of cancer care. We have been delighted with the success of this project so far, and we have only just begun.

REFERENCES

Aron, L., & Lechich, M. L. (2012). Relational psychoanalysis. In G. O. Gabbard, B. E. Litowitz, & P. Williams (Eds.), *Textbook of psychoanalysis* (2nd ed., pp. 211–224). American Psychiatric Publishing.

Caruso, R., Nanni, M. G., Rodin, G., Hales, S., Malfitano, C., De Padova, S., Bertelli, T., Belvederi Murri, M., Bovero, A., Miniotti, M., Leombruni, P., Zerbinati, L., Sabato, S., & Grassi, L. (2020). Effectiveness of a brief manualized intervention, Managing Cancer and Living Meaningfully (CALM), adapted to the Italian cancer care setting: Study protocol for a single-blinded randomized controlled trial. *Contemporary Clinical Trials Communications.* 2020 Oct 10; 20:100661. doi: 10.1016/j.conctc.2020.100661. eCollection 2020 Dec.

Caruso, R., Sabato, S., Nanni, M. G., Hales, S., Rodin, G., Malfitano, C., Tiberto, E., De Padova, S., Bertelli, T., Belvederi Murri, M., Zerbinati, L., & Grassi, L. (2020). Application of Managing Cancer and Living Meaningfully (CALM) in advanced cancer patients: An Italian pilot study. *Psychotherapy and Psychosomatics, 89*(6), 402–404.

de Vries, F. E., Mah, K., Shapiro, G. K., Rydall, A., Hales, S., & Rodin, G. (2020). Assessing the process of a brief psychotherapy for patients with advanced cancer. (Submitted for publication).

Engelmann, D., Scheffold, K., Friedrich, M., Hartung, T. J., Schulz-Kindermann, F., Lordick, F., Schilling, G., Lo, C., Rodin, G., & Mehnert, A. (2016). Death-related anxiety in patients with advanced cancer: Validation of the German version of the Death and Dying Distress Scale. *Journal of Pain and Symptom Management, 52*(4), 582–587.

Koranyi, S., Philipp, R., Quintero Garzón, L., Scheffold. K., Schulz-Kindermann, F., Härter, M., Rodin, G., Mehnert-Theuerkauf, A. (2020). Testing the treatment integrity of the Managing Cancer and Living Meaningfully psychotherapeutic intervention for patients with advanced cancer. *Frontiers in Psychology.* 2020 Dec 3;11:561997. doi: 10.3389/fpsyg.2020.561997. eCollection 2020.

Lo, C., Hales, S., Chiu, A., Panday, T., Malfitano, C., Jung, J., Rydall, A., Li, M., Nissim, R., Zimmermann, C., & Rodin, G. (2019). Managing Cancer And Living Meaningfully (CALM): Randomised feasibility trial in patients with advanced cancer. *BMJ Supportive & Palliative Care,* 9(2), 209–218. doi: 10.1136/bmjspcare-2015-000866. [Epub 2016 Jan 19].

Lo, C., Hales, S., Jung, J., Chiu, A., Panday, T., Rydall, A., Nissim, R., Malfitano, C., Petricone-Westwood, D., Zimmermann, C., & Rodin, G. (2014). Managing Cancer And Living Meaningfully (CALM): Phase 2 trial of a brief individual psychotherapy for patients with advanced cancer. *Palliative Medicine,* 28(3), 234–242.

Mehnert, A., Koranyi, S., Philipp, R., Scheffold, F., Kriston, L., Lehmann-Laue, A., Engelmann, D., Vehling, S., Eisenecker, C., Oechsle, K., Schulz-Kindermann, F., Rodin, G., & Härter, M. (2020). Efficacy of the Managing Cancer and Living Meaningfully (CALM) individual psychotherapy for patients with advanced cancer: A single-blind randomized controlled trial. *Psycho-Oncology,* 29(11), 1895–1904.

Nissim, R., Freeman, E., Lo, C., Zimmermann, C., Gagliese, L., Rydall, A., Hales, S., Rodin, G. (2012). Managing Cancer and Living Meaningfully (CALM): A qualitative study of a brief individual psychotherapy for individuals with advanced cancer. *Palliative Medicine,* 26(5), 713–721.

Rodin, G., Hales, S., & Lo, C. (Copyright 2015). *Managing Cancer And Living Meaningfully (CALM) Treatment Manual: An individual psychotherapy for patients with advanced disease.* Canadian Intellectual Property Office. Date of issue: 2015-09-04. Filing date: 2015-09-04; Copyright#: 1124205.

Rodin, G., Lo, C., Rydall, A., Shnall, J., Malfitano, C., Chiu, A., Panday, T., Watt, S., An, E., Nissim, R., Li, M., Zimmermann, C., & Hales, S. (2018). Managing Cancer and Living Meaningfully (CALM): A randomized controlled trial of a psychological intervention for patients with advanced cancer. *Journal of Clinical Oncology,* 36(23), 2422–2432.

Scheffold, K., Engelmann, D., Schulz-Kindermann, F., Rosenberger, C., Krüger, A., Rodin, G., Härter, M., & Mehnert, A. (2017). Managing cancer and living meaningfully: Qualitative pilot results of a sense-based short-term therapy for advanced cancer patients (CALM). *Psychotherapeut,* 62, 243–248.

Scheffold, K., Philipp, R., Engelmann, D., Schulz-Kindermann, F., Rosenberger, C., Oechsle, K., Härter, M., Wegscheider, K., Lordick, F., Lo, C., Hales, S., Rodin, G., & Mehnert, A. (2015). Efficacy of a brief manualized intervention Managing Cancer and Living Meaningfully (CALM) adapted to German cancer care settings: Study protocol for a randomized controlled trial. *BMC Cancer,* 15(1), 592. doi: 10.1186/s12885-015-1589-y.

Scheffold, K., Wollbrück, D., Schulz-Kindermann, F., Rosenberger, C., Krüger, A., Lo, C., Hales, S., Rodin, G., Härter, M., & Mehnert, A. (2015). Pilot results of the German Managing Cancer and Living Meaningfully (CALM) RCT: A brief individual psychotherapy for advanced cancer patients. *BMC Cancer,* 15, 592.

Statistics Canada. (2019a, August 9). *Census profile, 2016 census.* https://www12.statcan.gc.ca/census-recensement/2016/dp-pd/prof/details/page.cfm?Lang=E

&Geo1=CSD&Code1=3520005&Geo2=CD&Code2=3520&SearchText=Toronto
&SearchType=Begins&SearchPR=01&B1=All&TABID=1&type=0

Statistics Canada. (2019b, June 19). *Focus on geography series, 2016 Census.* https://
www12.statcan.gc.ca/census-recensement/2016/as-sa/fogs-spg/Facts-CSD-
eng.cfm?TOPIC=7&LANG=eng&GK=CSD&GC=3520005

Troncoso, P., Rydall, A., Hales, S., & Rodin, G. (2019). A review of psychosocial
interventions in patients with advanced cancer in Latin America and the
value of CALM therapy in this setting. *American Journal of Psychiatry and
Neuroscience*, 7(4), 108–118.

Tseng, W. S. (2001). *Handbook of cultural psychiatry*. Academic Press.

PART 2
The CALM Treatment Manual

MANUAL INTRODUCTION

Putting the essential elements of therapy into words encourages clarity but also risks eliminating or ignoring the human and creative dimensions of the therapeutic process. Many key therapeutic elements—what we feel with our patients, our focused interest and attention, and our ability to understand our individual patients—are difficult to capture in a manual. Nevertheless, treatment manuals that define and illustrate the essential dimensions of an intervention enhance the rigor of psychotherapeutic research and help to ensure the reliability of treatment delivery. In the following chapters, we describe the essential elements of Managing Cancer and Living Meaningfully (CALM). We hope that we have left room for the human and imaginative capacities of patients and therapists and for the adaptation of CALM to different settings, populations, cultures, and languages.

Some of the features of CALM described in the chapters that follow are common to many therapies; some are even the specific focus of other therapeutic approaches. This manual is intended to capture these common therapeutic elements while also highlighting what is unique and specific about CALM. To some extent, CALM can be regarded as an assemblage of techniques and approaches, in that its specificity and uniqueness derive primarily from the ways in which the content and process are organized. As described in a recent commission on the integration of palliative care in oncology (Kaasa et al., 2018), CALM is intended to be integrated with both cancer care and palliative care to provide patients with advanced disease and their caregivers the reflective space to communicate their experiences and to address the major decisions, burdens, and adaptive challenges of advanced and progressive disease.

While Part I of this book explains the theoretical and empirical foundations of CALM, Part II is an operational guide or manual for clinicians and researchers to ensure the integrity and fidelity of CALM delivered in different settings. Such a guide is needed for CALM to be delivered as intended in different parts of the world and for research outcomes in diverse settings to be meaningfully compared.

This manual is intended as a tool for therapists-in-training and as a reference for trained therapists. For those beginning their reading with Part II of this book, the manual first provides a brief review of the background and structure of CALM. It then explains and illustrates the essential elements of CALM delivery. Note, however, that this guide is not meant to replace the didactic and clinical training that is required for therapists to become competent in this modality.

This book and the manual within it has been, in some respects, more than a decade in the making. The first CALM manual was developed as part of the protocol of our initial CALM pilot study. We have since deepened our thinking through the many grant applications and publications that we have composed and through the presentations and workshops that we have delivered. Our experiences with our patients and our colleagues locally and around the world have also pushed us to elaborate and refine our thinking about CALM. As a consequence, we came to feel that there should be a place where it could all be put together. We hope that this manual will serve this purpose and act as a guidebook or map to the landscape of CALM, although we recognize that there is so much more we have yet to see and understand.

REFERENCE

Kaasa, S., Loge, J. H., Aapro, M., Albreht, T., Anderson, R., Bruera, E., Brunelli, C., Caraceni, A., Cervantes, A., Currow, D. C., Deliens, L., Fallon, M., Gómez-Batiste, X., Grotmol, K. S., Hannon, B., Haugen, D. F., Higginson, I. J., Hjermstad, M. J., Hui, D., Jordan, K., Kurita, G. P., Larkin, P. J., Miccinesi, G., Nauck, F., Pribakovic, R., Rodin, G., Sjøgren, P., Stone, P., Zimmermann, C., & Lundeby, T. (2018). Integration of oncology and palliative care: A Lancet Oncology Commission. *The Lancet Oncology*, *19*(11), e588–e653. doi: 10.1016/S1470-2045(18)30415-7.

CHAPTER 13

Rationale, Foundations, and Goals of CALM

INTRODUCTION

For those who come first to the manual, the following text provides a brief overview of the rationale for Managing Cancer and Living Meaningfully (CALM) therapy and the foundations on which it was built. It also introduces the overarching goals of the CALM intervention.

RATIONALE FOR CALM

The onset, progression, or recurrence of serious or advanced disease may trigger an acute grief reaction, including feelings of shock, disbelief, emotional numbness, and denial of the objective reality of the illness. However, the initial and subsequent responses of a person to the diagnosis and course of advanced disease depends on their psychological organizing principles, the nature and personal meaning of the disease, and their prior experience with illness and other traumatic events. Feelings of sadness, loss, defectiveness, isolation, and helplessness are common, as is damage to the sense of identity and personal value. Even those who have been previously well adjusted and without prior psychiatric or psychological vulnerability may experience severe emotional distress in the wake of serious illness and its effects. Anxiety is the most common initial psychological symptom of distress following the diagnosis of advanced disease (Gurevich et al., 2002;

see Chapter 2 of this volume). Depression is more frequent with disease progression and proximity to death (Lo et al., 2010) and may be regarded as a final common pathway of distress, dependent on the interaction between the multiple stressors of advanced disease and individual strengths and vulnerabilities (Rodin et al., 2009).

Psychotherapy is a fundamental treatment modality to relieve distress and promote well-being in individuals with advanced disease. The circumstance of advanced illness and the threat of impending mortality may facilitate and deepen the psychotherapeutic process for a number of reasons. The distress and disequilibrium caused by the onset of metastatic cancer may heighten the motivation and need for psychological support. The perceived shortness of time may also create a heightened sense of urgency to address important issues. Finally, there is typically an exquisite desire for authenticity that may facilitate and deepen the therapeutic relationship.

THE FOUNDATIONS OF CALM

CALM is rooted in several broad theoretical traditions, including self-psychology, relational theory, attachment theory, and existential theory. Self-psychology posits that the self, defined as the continuity of subjective experience, is the central structure of the mind and that the organization and consolidation of subjective experience is the central psychotherapeutic task (Kohut, 1977). Relational theory emphasizes the bidirectional nature of the therapeutic situation in which the patient and therapist co-create meaning and understanding of the patient's experience (Mitchell, 1988). Attachment theory posits that early experiences with caregivers consolidate internalized cognitive schemas, or working models, of the self in relation to others that shape the sense of connection to others and the capacity to seek, accept, or make use of support (Bowlby, 1969, 1973, 1980). Attachment security refers to the tendency of individuals to believe that they are worthy of care and that others are trustworthy to provide it. The onset of disease activates the attachment system, heightening the importance and salience of attachment security and the fears that it may not be available (see Chapter 4 of this volume). A psychotherapeutic relationship may enhance attachment security and facilitate adjustment to the radical alterations in attachment needs that occur in those with advanced disease.

Existential psychotherapy (Yalom, 1980) is an approach rooted in the analytic and humanist traditions and influenced by existential philosophy.

It is concerned with the conflicts that arise when individuals confront the inescapable human challenges of death, relatedness, autonomy, and meaning. The psychotherapeutic process of CALM can help individuals manage and tolerate the emotional distress that arises from this confrontation and can support psychological growth and development at this late stage of life.

CALM also draws upon other manualized psychotherapeutic interventions that have been developed to alleviate distress and support meaning-making in those with advanced and life-threatening illness (see Chapter 9 of this volume). These include supportive-expressive group therapy (Classen et al., 2001; Goodwin et al., 2001; Spiegel et al., 1981), cognitive existential group therapy (Kissane et al., 2003, 2004), and meaning-centered individual and group psychotherapy (Breitbart et al., 2004). These approaches were developed as interventions focused on existential, spiritual, or meaning-centered issues pertinent to this population. Dignity Therapy (Chochinov et al., 2005) is an individual intervention designed to enhance meaning and the sense of a positive legacy for individuals near the end of life. By design, CALM is broader in scope and aim than these interventions. It is intended to address the practical, relational, and existential challenges that arise for those with advanced disease while helping them remain engaged with life. The goal of CALM is to support both the living and dying processes. We term the capacity to sustain this duality as "double awareness" (Rodin & Zimmermann, 2008).

THE OVERARCHING GOALS OF CALM

The reduction and prevention of psychological distress and support for "double awareness" are primary goals of CALM that are achieved by providing relational support, help with affect regulation, and the opportunity for patients to reflect on the domains of experience that are relevant to their situation. These domains have been conceptualized in CALM as:

1. Collaboration and negotiation with healthcare providers to support decision-making and optimize cancer care and symptom control;
2. Adjustments in the sense of identity and renegotiation of attachment relationships with spouses, families, and significant others in the new context of the disease;
3. Review and reprioritization of the sources of meaning and purpose in life; and
4. Fears, hopes, and concerns about the future and about mortality.

Although the symptomatic relief of distress is an important goal of CALM, the intervention is also intended to support psychological growth and development. This is consistent with Erikson's (1982) view that psychological growth can occur in the last stage of life with the attainment of wisdom. His definition of wisdom as "the informed and detached concern for life itself in the face of death itself" (p. 61) has much in common with our concept of double awareness (Rodin & Zimmermann, 2008). Colarusso (1992) applied Spitz's (1965) concept of "psychic organizer" to refer to the powerful effect that an awareness of the shortness of time has on the motivation to reflect on the life that has been lived and is yet to be lived. This is consistent with other research that has examined the potential for posttraumatic growth following trauma, including that associated with cancer and other life-threatening illnesses (see Chapter 8 of this volume). Taken together, these views suggest that life-threatening illness may precipitate a developmental crisis that, in turn, may initiate creative change and growth.

CONCLUSION

CALM was developed based on the theoretical foundations of relational, attachment, and existential theory and upon earlier psychotherapeutic approaches. Intended to be integrated with cancer care and palliative care, CALM aims to help patients with advanced cancer live their lives as well as possible while also facing the challenges of their disease and treatment. This is achieved by providing relational support, help with affect regulation, and the opportunity to reflect on the four CALM domains.

REFERENCES

Bowlby, J. (1969). *Attachment and loss*. Vol. 1: *Attachment*. Hogarth Press and the Institute of Psycho-Analysis.

Bowlby, J. (1973). *Attachment and loss*. Vol. 2: *Separation, anxiety and anger*. Hogarth Press and the Institute of Psycho-Analysis.

Bowlby, J. (1980). *Attachment and loss*. Vol. 3: *Loss: Sadness and depression*. Hogarth Press and Institute of Psycho-Analysis.

Breitbart, W., Gibson, C., Poppito, S. R., & Berg, A. (2004). Psychotherapeutic interventions at the end of life: A focus on meaning and spirituality. *Canadian Journal of Psychiatry, 49*(6), 366–372.

Chochinov, H. M., Hack, T., Hassard, T., Kristjanson, L. J., McClement, S., & Harlos, M. (2005). Dignity therapy: A novel psychotherapeutic intervention for patients near the end of life. *Journal of Clinical Oncology, 23*(24), 5520–5525.

Classen, C., Butler, L. D., Koopman, C., Miller, E., DiMiceli, S., Giese-Davis, J., Fobair, P., Carlson, R. W., Kraemer, H. C, & Spiegel, D. (2001). Supportive-expressive group therapy and distress in patients with metastatic breast cancer: A randomized clinical intervention trial. *Archives of General Psychiatry, 58*(5), 494–501.

Colarusso, C. A. (1992). *Child and adult development: A psychoanalytic introduction for clinicians*. Springer Science+Business Media New York.

Erikson, E. H. (1982). *The life cycle completed*. W. W. Norton & Company.

Goodwin, P. J., Leszcz, M., Ennis, M., Koopmans, J., Vincent, L., Guther, H., Drysdale, E., Hundleby, M., Chochinov, H. M., Navarro, M., Speca, M., Masterson, J., Dohan, L., Sela, R., Warren, B., Paterson, A., Pritchard, K. I., Arnold, A., Doll, R., O'Reilly, S. E., Quirt, G., Hood, N., & Hunter, J. (2001). The effect of group psychosocial support on survival in metastatic breast cancer. *The New England Journal of Medicine, 345*(24), 1719–1726.

Gurevich, M., Devins, G. M., & Rodin, G. M. (2002). Stress response syndromes and cancer: Conceptual and assessment issues. *Psychosomatics, 43*(4), 259–281.

Kissane, D. W., Bloch, S., Smith, G. C., Miach, P., Clarke, D. M., Ikin, J., Love, A., Ranieri, N., & McKenzie, D. (2003). Cognitive-existential group psychotherapy for women with primary breast cancer: A randomised controlled trial. *Psycho-Oncology, 12*(6), 532–546.

Kissane, D. W., Love, A., Hatton, A., Bloch, S., Smith, G., Clarke, D. M., Miach, P., Ikin, J., Ranieri, N., & Snyder, R. D. (2004). Effect of cognitive-existential group therapy on survival in early-stage breast cancer. *Journal of Clinical Oncology, 22*(21), 4255–4260.

Kohut, H. (1977). *The restoration of the self*. International Universities Press.

Lo, C., Zimmermann, C., Rydall, A., Walsh, A., Jones, J. M., Moore, M. J., Shepherd, F.A., Gagliese, L., & Rodin, G. (2010). Longitudinal study of depressive symptoms in patients with metastatic gastrointestinal and lung cancer. *Journal of Clinical Oncology, 28*(18), 3084–3089.

Mitchell, S. A. (1988). *Relational concepts in psychoanalysis: An integration*. Harvard University Press.

Rodin, G., Lo, C., Mikulincer, M., Donner, A., Gagliese, L., & Zimmermann, C. (2009). Pathways to distress: The multiple determinants of depression, hopelessness and the desire for hastened death in metastatic cancer patients. *Social Science & Medicine, 68*(3), 562–569.

Rodin, G., & Zimmermann, C. (2008). Psychoanalytic reflections on mortality: A reconsideration. *Journal of the American Academy of Psychoanalysis and Dynamic Psychiatry, 36*(1), 181–196.

Spiegel, D., Bloom, J. R., & Yalom, I. D. (1981). Group support for patients with metastatic cancer: A randomized outcome study. *Archives of General Psychiatry, 38*(5), 527–533.

Spitz, R. A. (1965). *The first year of life: A psychoanalytic study of normal and deviant development of object relations*. International Universities Press.

Yalom, I. D. (1980). *Existential psychotherapy*. Basic Books.

CHAPTER 14

The Structure and Process of CALM

INTRODUCTION

The following text describes the characteristics of both patients and therapists that tend to foster success in CALM therapy and outlines the format, session tasks, and process of the CALM intervention.

THE SUITABLE PATIENT

CALM was designed for patients with advanced or life-threatening cancer who are motivated to receive psychological help and are willing and able to engage in a process that involves introspection and the expression of feelings. Typically, patients must be well enough physically and cognitively to engage in sessions of approximately 45 minutes in length. CALM is brief, usually three to six sessions delivered over a three- to six-month period, and is most beneficial if there is a period of wellness anticipated in the patient's disease trajectory to allow for therapy completion. The optimal timing of CALM is variable, as patients who are newly diagnosed may not yet have understood the meaning of their illness and their attention may be focused on immediate treatment decisions. The most common point at which patients are motivated to receive CALM is when they perceive that they are at a "tipping point"—often when treatments have failed to halt progression of their disease or when new debilitating symptoms emerge. At such times, there is often heightened distress, fears associated with mortality, and great adjustments that must be made. The potential benefits of CALM are more limited if it is initiated late in the course of the disease when patients may be too unwell to participate and when opportunities to be engaged in life have diminished.

CALM is intended to help patients make sense of their illness experience. This approach is consistent with evidence that understanding ourselves and our current circumstance from a longitudinal perspective, referred to as autobiographical reasoning, allows us to create a history that can be shared and helps us manage difficult life events (Habermas, 2011; Weststrate & Glück, 2017). Participation in CALM requires some interest in or capacity for psychological understanding, which is captured in the concept of mentalization (see Chapter 5 of this volume), although there can be considerable variation in the ability or motivation to engage in this. Mentalization is operationalized as reflective functioning and refers to the interest or capacity of individuals to accept that there can be multiple perspectives on events and experiences and to reflect on their own subjective state and that of others (Jurist, 2010). Although mentalization has often been viewed as an individual capacity, it is also a process that emerges within relationships, including those with a therapist (Shaw et al., 2020).

The patient-identified caregiver is invited to one or more CALM sessions to explore couple or family functioning in the face of advanced disease. This brings another perspective into the sessions and allows the therapist to observe and improve couple communication, mutual understanding, and the capacity to work collaboratively to manage the challenges of the disease and its treatment. Solely individual CALM sessions may be required when the patient declines to invite a caregiver and/or when the caregiver is unavailable or unwilling to be constructively engaged or cannot tolerate the communication of distress and the reflective process.

THE CALM THERAPIST

Therapeutic encounters with patients with advanced disease may be some of the most intimate and profound of all therapeutic relationships. The universality and the inescapability of the dilemma facing those with advanced disease brings poignancy to the interaction and often creates an intimate bond between patient and therapist. Indeed, accepting the shared experience of human mortality may be a prerequisite for therapists to immerse themselves in the emotional world of those living with advanced disease. The quality of the therapeutic relationship is a central element in most psychotherapies but is particularly important in the therapy of patients with advanced and life-threatening illness because of their level of distress and their need for empathic attunement, genuineness, and the emotional presence of the therapist.

The engagement of the CALM therapist may allow the patient to be understood in an experience-near fashion, which may be deeply and positively meaningful for both parties. This has much in common with what composer Pauline Oliveros described as deep listening that "digs below the surface of what is heard . . . unlocking layer after layer of imagination, meaning and memory" (as cited in Pavlicevic & Impey, 2013, p. 238). Listening in this way may trigger a wide range of experiences in the therapist, including feelings of grief, guilt, sorrow, detachment, and reflections about mortality and the sense of meaning and purpose in life. Attending to their own inner life in this situation may be a unique pathway for therapists to understand the experience of the patient and create a new shared experience. This so-called analytic third (Ogden, 2004) may then transform the individual subjectivities of both parties. Regular CALM supervision is important and recommended for those engaged in CALM therapy to enhance these skills and manage this process.

CALM is best delivered in the context of holistic cancer care, where adequate attention is also given to pain and symptom relief, psychopharmacological interventions, caregiver burden, and advance care planning. CALM training has been successfully provided to professionals from a wide range of health disciplines that include psychotherapeutic care within their scope of practice, including palliative care physicians, oncologists, psychologists, psychiatrists, nurses, social workers, and spiritual care providers. Patients report benefit from working with a therapist who is an "insider" into the world of cancer care, who understands treatment protocols and terminology, and who is familiar with the course of disease and its practical challenges.

THE FORMAT

CALM therapy consists of three to six individual or couple-based sessions of approximately 45 minutes delivered over three to six months. The timing and duration of these sessions can vary based on the needs of the patient and the clinical course of the disease and treatment. The four domains of CALM represent the general content themes that patients are given an opportunity to reflect upon at some point over the course of the intervention (see Chapter 15 of this volume). These domains need not necessarily receive equal time and attention, nor are they considered mutually exclusive. They are meant to provide a general framework for therapists to keep in mind regarding the issues and concerns that are likely to be relevant to patients with advanced disease and their partners and families.

GENERAL SESSION TASKS AND GUIDELINES

The tasks of the first session are to: (a) introduce the patient to the overall goals of the intervention, the content of the domains, and the nature of the therapeutic process; (b) gather background information that will inform the therapist about the personal history of the patient, the trajectory of the disease, and the nature of their current symptoms and concerns; and (c) establish a therapeutic relationship and atmosphere in which the patient can speak openly about his or her feelings and in which there is opportunity for reflection (see CALM Session 1 Therapy Notes in Appendix G). The general guideline for the first session includes:

- Collection of background information (age, gender, sexual identity, marital and living arrangements, cultural background and identity, constellation of immediate family members and close personal relationships, current and past employment, and sources of financial and practical support).
- Review of current psychological distress, well-being, health status, practical support, and coping strategies.
- Encouragement of the patient to tell the story of the disease from the onset of symptoms to the cancer diagnosis, treatment, course of the disease, and understanding of the future course.
- A brief medical history and psychiatric history, including past psychiatric diagnoses, treatments including other forms of psychotherapy and counseling, hospitalizations, self-harm and suicidality, aggression, and substance use.
- Obtaining a personal and developmental history that includes information about early family life, childhood, identity, and relational functioning.
- Introduction to CALM goals and organization and brief review of the four domains.
- Provision of an initial agreed upon understanding of the patient in their context and the goals for future sessions.
- Discussion of the tentative treatment plan, including the number of sessions and scheduling for following sessions.
- Invitation to bring a primary family caregiver, if they have not already joined the first session, to come to at least one session that will

be devoted to relational aspects of living with cancer. In some cases, spouses or other family members will attend all CALM sessions. Such joint sessions are most likely to be desirable and productive when there is a close and collaborative relationship prior to the onset of the disease, when relational issues are the patient's primary concern, and/or when both parties can tolerate the communication of distressing feelings.

The middle sessions are intended to provide a supportive atmosphere in which patients can speak openly about their feelings, explore in greater depth the four CALM content domains, and promote mentalization to facilitate double awareness (see CALM Sessions 2–8 Therapy Notes in Appendix H). A general guideline for the middle sessions includes:

- A review of current psychological distress, well-being, health status, and the patient's experience in therapy and in communicating emotional distress.
- An exploration of the patient's experience as it relates to the four domains. This includes:
  - Discussion of relationships with healthcare providers and treatment decisions.
  - Review of attachment relationships and renegotiation of attachment relationships that has occurred or is needed.
  - Review of current sources of satisfaction and meaning.
  - Discussion about advance care planning and exploration of distress about dying and death.

The task of the final session is to reflect on the CALM therapy, the adjustments that have occurred, and the challenges and tasks that may lie ahead. A general guideline for this session includes:

- A review of level of psychological distress, well-being, and health status.
- A summary of the important themes that have emerged and how the patient has addressed these issues.
- An exploration of feelings related to the end of the therapy.
- An invitation to contact the therapist for additional sessions as the need might arise.

It should be noted that many CALM therapies do not end with a formal last session. When there is a plateau in the disease course, the therapy may be paused with the understanding that it can resume when there is another "tipping point" in the progression of the disease. In other cases, a patient may become unwell and unable to return for a final session. The potential lack of closure may be a lost and missed opportunity that both the patient and therapist may experience.

THE PROCESS

CALM is intended to create space for patients to reflect on the four specified domains, however the process is individualized to meet the changing needs of the patient, family, and the moment in therapy. An overall therapeutic strategy is to facilitate mentalization, which is the capacity to reflect on feeling states, to distinguish them from literal facts, and to accept the possibility of multiple perspectives on events. This may be particularly important in the face of mortality to sustain and tolerate "double awareness" (Rodin & Zimmermann, 2008) with the contemplation of and planning for disease progression, while also maintaining engagement with life. This capacity is facilitated when the therapeutic relationship provides a secure base for patients and families.

There are a number of active ingredients of CALM that may contribute to its therapeutic effect, some of which are shared with other psychotherapeutic modalities. It is the assemblage of these ingredients, along with attention to the CALM domains, that is unique to CALM. These ingredients are:

1. *The supportive relationship*. An empathic understanding of and appreciation for the patient's felt experience is a foundation of CALM. Through this, the therapist becomes a witness to the patient's journey, decreasing their sense of isolation, helping them to identify strengths, and encouraging the use of adaptive coping strategies.
2. *Authenticity*. The therapeutic stance in CALM is one of genuineness and honesty in relation to the patient, encouraging and modeling a similar stance in the patient. Experience and judgment are required to maintain professional boundaries while sustaining a posture of mutual engagement. Therapists must navigate this balance when deciding how to respond to personal questions that may arise, such as "Do you believe in God?" or "Have you faced death in your immediate family?"
3. *Modulation of affect*. By attending to the emotional state of the patient and demonstrating comfort with emotional distress, the therapist may help the patient to build confidence and a greater capacity to manage emotions. The intent is to support emotional communication and to protect patients from emotional hyperarousal or emotional detachment

and numbing. This was important for a woman with ovarian cancer and posttraumatic stress symptoms who experienced intense and overwhelming affect states that interfered with her capacity to think and reflect both within and outside of CALM sessions. The engagement of the therapist had a calming effect that diminished her distressing state of isolation and increased her capacity to maintain affect states within a window of tolerability. In other cases, the therapist may enhance the capacity of patients and their partners to share their emotional experiences, to absorb the distress of the other, and to become a more effective system of mutual influence (Lo et al., 2013).

4. *Renegotiation of attachment security.* The relational adjustments imposed by the disease and the distress related to these changes are explored in CALM. A deepening of spousal relationships often occurs, but there may also be disequilibrium in these relationships in response to heightened dependency needs and the patient's diminished capacity for autonomy. Individuals who have tended to be self-sufficient and/or comfortable in the caregiving role, typical of those with a so-called avoidant attachment style, may be threatened by the growing dependency necessitated by progressive disease. Whereas those who are anxiously attached may experience increasing fear about the loss of support, the avoidantly attached may become deeply distressed about the loss of their capacity for autonomy and their need to depend on others. These changes trigger disequilibrium in important relationships and create an urgent need to adjust and renegotiate the terms of these relationships to regain attachment security.

    For a middle-aged man with progressive thymic cancer, his diminished strength and self-sufficiency had stimulated deeply disturbing feelings of dependency. His initial response to his increasing weakness and reliance on others was to become more controlling of his wife, who reacted with withdrawal. The CALM treatment process allowed this man to mourn the loss of his previous strength and to express his needs more openly to his wife. She responded positively to this expression of need and to his validation of her caregiving. The long prior history of positive feelings between them allowed a renegotiation of their relationship based on their current attachment needs.

5. *The joint creation of meaning.* The meanings that patients have attached to their life history, to their perceived accomplishments and failures, and to the challenges in the context of illness are explored in CALM sessions. The therapist may be able to validate their sense of pride in their accomplishments in the domains of family, work, or the community and acknowledge disappointments or regrets. The latter may

involve goals or plans that might now never be achieved or problematic relationships in the past or present that may never be fixed. New meanings or possibilities may also emerge in the dialogue regarding the patient's life trajectory, goals, the suffering associated with the disease, and the end of life. The therapist may be able to collaborate with the patient to create new meanings for the past, present, or future life that may bring greater acceptance or equanimity. The ability and willingness to explore these questions are facilitated by a growing capacity to tolerate emotions, which may be enabled by CALM.

6. *Shifting frame and flexibility.* Fluctuations in the patient's clinical state, symptom control, and the receipt of prognostic news may drastically alter the capacity or motivation for self-reflection. This may necessitate shifts in therapeutic goals and adjustment of the content and timing of sessions based on the patient's physical state and concurrent medical treatments. Emotional exploration may be less feasible or may even be contraindicated when patients are experiencing severe pain or anxiety or are in the midst of a medical crisis. At such times, the therapeutic focus should be to bolster adaptive coping strategies and to maintain psychological equilibrium. This was evident in a woman with advanced cancer in whom the development of brain metastases triggered a flood of intense emotions and a frightening awareness of her mortality and the young children she would leave behind. The therapist shifted to a more supportive mode, with a focus on managing intolerable affect and attachment security.

7. *Facing the therapeutic limits and boundaries.* The willingness of therapists to face the unsettling topics of mortality and suffering may allow patients to do the same in the sessions. The deep engagement of therapists in this process requires them to face their own fears of mortality and suffering and to accept the limits of their therapeutic influence on the outcome of the disease. The therapeutic goal in this circumstance is to allow expression of sadness and anxiety about the progression of disease and the confrontation with morality, while also sustaining hope, morale, and engagement in the present. In some cases, this may involve accepting the impossibility of achieving life goals that had seemed vitally important. For a couple who had devoted themselves to work in the hope that retirement would bring freedom and the opportunity to travel, the diagnosis and progression of metastatic prostate cancer meant relinquishing this goal and living with inescapable disappointment and regret. These feelings were profound and associated with a kind of paralysis in making any other plans. The CALM therapist helped them to reconsider possibilities for the future and to reframe goals that might still be

achievable, reflecting a kind of double awareness. Another woman with metastatic gastrointestinal cancer felt locked into an unhappy marriage with a disengaged husband who had developed an intimate relationship with another woman. CALM helped her tolerate this unchangeable situation and find alternative sources of support at this most difficult time in her life.

8. *Interpretation.* Interpretations in psychodynamic therapy were traditionally considered to be explanations provided by the therapist about the meaning of the patient's symptoms or behavior. In more recent years, the process of interpretation has come to be understood as a joint creation of meaning that is made possible by a "meeting of the minds" (Aron, 1996), arising from immersion in the patient's experience and the dialogue between patient and therapist. These interpretations are offered tentatively and in the spirit of collaboration. Such a process may allow patients to understand themselves more deeply and to consider alternative ways of thinking and feeling about themselves and their situation. In that regard, a female professional with metastatic breast cancer who had grown up being a "good girl" who always felt she should meet the expectations of others now felt a sense of shame and embarrassment that her illness would disappoint those around her. Understanding that her beliefs reflected a way of thinking that did not necessarily correspond to what others actually thought or expected had a liberating effect. Interpretations made in this way help to expand awareness and consideration of alternate ways of thinking, reflecting the process of mentalization described next and in Chapter 5 of this volume.

9. *Mentalization and "double awareness."* Individuals vary widely in their capacity for self-reflection and mentalization. These terms refer to the capacity to reflect on feeling states, to distinguish them from literal facts, and to accept the possibility of multiple perspectives. Sustaining the capacity to mentalize is a particular challenge in the context of advanced disease because the reality of the disease and the literal threat of impending mortality may obscure the understanding that hopelessness or demoralization are mental constructs, or only one of multiple ways that their situation can be viewed. The mentalization of such feelings can allow individuals with advanced disease to sustain a "double awareness" of the possibilities for living as well as the eventuality of dying. The CALM therapist promotes this by understanding and validating the experience of the patient while also entertaining the possibility of multiple psychological responses to an incontrovertibly dire prognosis. Paradoxically, identifying the unique and personal meaning

of the illness can highlight that other ways of thinking and feeling are possible.

10. *Endings*. Most patients who engage in CALM complete three to six sessions. Such individuals often do not want longer term therapy, although the duration of CALM may be prolonged when there are ongoing crises or may be paused when the disease is in a stable, more chronic phase. In many cases, the timing of the final CALM session is mutually decided upon by the patient and therapist, with patients invited to return to the therapist in the future as needed. Structuring treatment to include time to say farewell is important in some cases but should arise from the patient's wishes and be conducted with the understanding that goodbye does not signify "giving up" or that subsequent sessions are not possible. In many cases, there is no formal end or termination of therapy because death or the rapid progression of disease may occur unexpectedly. One patient with metastatic prostate cancer who feared such an abrupt end likened his situation to being in an old Western movie where "the wagons were circled and we were surrounded." Discussion of these concerns may be therapeutic and sessions that are productive and engaging may occur very near to a patient's death.

CONCLUSION

This chapter describes the structure of CALM, its format, and the essential ingredients of the therapeutic process. Integrating these themes and elements and tailoring them to the fluctuating needs of individual patients and couples are skills that are supported by CALM training and supervision.

REFERENCES

Aron, L. (1996). *A meeting of minds: Mutuality in psychoanalysis*. Relational Perspectives Book Series 4. The Analytic Press.

Habermas, T. (2011). Autobiographical reasoning: Arguing and narrating from a biographical perspective. *New Directions for Child and Adolescent Development, 2011*(131), 1–17.

Jurist, E. L. (2010). Mentalizing minds. *Psychoanalytic Inquiry, 30*(4), 289–300.

Lo, C., Hales, S., Braun, M., Rydall, A. C., Zimmermann, C., & Rodin, G. (2013). Couples facing advanced cancer: Examination of an interdependent relational system. *Psycho-Oncology, 22*(10), 2283–2290.

Ogden, T. H. (2004). The analytic third: Implications for psychoanalytic theory and technique. *The Psychoanalytic Quarterly, 73*(1), 167–195.

Pavlicevic, M., & Impey, A. (2013). *Deep listening:* Towards an imaginative reframing of health and well-being practices in international development. *Arts & Health, 5*(3), 238–252.

Rodin, G., & Zimmermann, C. (2008). Psychoanalytic reflections on mortality: A reconsideration. *Journal of the American Academy of Psychoanalysis and Dynamic Psychiatry, 36*(1), 181–196.

Shaw, C., Lo, C., Lanceley, A., Hales, S., & Rodin, G. (2020). The assessment of mentalization: Measures for the patient, the therapist, and the interaction. *Journal of Contemporary Psychotherapy, 50*(1), 57–65. https:// doi.org/ 10.1007/ s10879- 019- 09420- z.

Weststrate, N. M., & Glück, J. (2017). Hard-earned wisdom: Exploratory processing of difficult life experience is positively associated with wisdom. *Developmental Psychology, 53*(4), 800–814.

CHAPTER 15
The CALM Domains

INTRODUCTION

The four domains described in this chapter represent the general content themes that all patients are given the opportunity to address during CALM. The initial interview is used to briefly explore each of these areas and to identify the domains that are most pressing or problematic. Each domain does not necessarily receive equal time and attention, nor are they mutually exclusive. The therapy often moves fluidly between these interrelated domains within and between sessions. After the initial three to six sessions, subsequent booster sessions can be offered as needed and can focus on the most relevant domain(s) at that time.

The goals in exploring each domain are provided next, with suggested prompts to initiate exploration of these content areas and case examples that combine domain content and therapeutic process elements.

DOMAIN 1: SYMPTOM MANAGEMENT AND COMMUNICATION WITH HEALTHCARE PROVIDERS

The general goals of this domain are to:

1. Empathically explore the patient's experience of symptoms, general functioning, and relationships with healthcare team members; and
2. Support and encourage the patient's active involvement in their medical care, including understanding their disease and forming collaborative

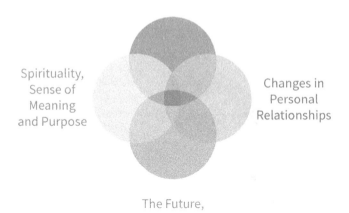

Symptom Management
and Communication with
Healthcare Providers

Spirituality,
Sense of
Meaning
and Purpose

Changes in
Personal
Relationships

The Future,
Hope and Mortality

Figure 15.1. The CALM domains
From "Managing Cancer and Living Meaningfully (CALM) Therapy," by S. Hales, C. Lo, and G. Rodin, in J. C. Holland, W. S. Breitbart, P. N. Butow, P. B. Jacobsen, M. J. Loscalzo, & R. McCorkle (Eds.), Psycho-Oncology (3rd ed., p. 487, Figure 62.1), 2015, Oxford University Press. © Oxford University Press 2015. Reproduced with permission of the Licensor through PLSclear.

relationships with healthcare providers to support symptom control and medical decision-making.

Suggested probes to initiate discussion:

- "Tell me the story of your cancer diagnosis and treatment to date."
- "How do you feel about the healthcare you have been receiving?"
- "What is the nature of your relationship with the medical team? Can you describe areas in which you are satisfied, and areas in which you may be less satisfied?"
- "To what extent can you communicate your questions and concerns to the medical team?" or "To what extent do you feel listened to by your medical team?"
- "How are you feeling physically these days?"
- "What do you understand about your current cancer treatment plan?"

Understanding the disease and managing symptoms: The process of understanding the disease and learning to manage it effectively takes time. Patients may benefit from help in understanding the information provided by physicians and other healthcare providers or obtained from other sources, such as from family, friends, and the internet. Addressing misunderstandings or cognitive distortions may be of particular value following the diagnosis of cancer or other serious medical conditions, since benign or coincidental physical symptoms or medical investigations commonly trigger profound anxiety and worry. Helping patients to distinguish symptoms that are likely to be related to the disease and its progression from those that are due to coincidental medical conditions or treatment toxicity may help relieve distress. Therapists may also play a role in helping patients reflect on the information that they wish to obtain from their healthcare providers, and particularly that which is related to understanding their disease status and treatment decisions.

Case Example 1

A woman with breast cancer metastatic to her bones had experienced recurrent bouts of significant anxiety and bone pain, often occurring together.

Patient: "I don't know what's wrong with me. I was doing so well and now I am feeling on edge and tearful. I have been experiencing a lot of pain in my left leg lately. I don't know why and I don't know what to do."

CALM therapeutic responses: "Who in your care team can you contact about this pain for further investigation and pain relief?" "What has made it difficult for you to let your medical team know about these symptoms?" Then, "You've told me, in the past, that your anxiety is often triggered by physical distress. What thoughts does this pain trigger in you?"

The therapeutic strategy is to help this patient consider how to manage her physical symptoms and to seek appropriate help for symptom relief. An additional goal is to explore the underlying meaning of these symptoms for her, which may include the fear that the disease is advancing, that she is dying, or that she will become disabled by pain and more dependent on caregivers. Such interventions may help the patient to feel understood and to consider alternative possibilities to manage both physical and psychological distress.

Non-CALM response: "You should call your radiation oncologist. They have been able to radiate and relieve your symptoms in the past. You may be worrying too much about this."

While the therapist may be intending to provide reassurance to decrease the patient's anxiety, this response could be experienced as silencing or dismissive of the patient's feelings and does not allow for further exploration or understanding of the cause of the emotional response. Further, problem-solving of this kind by the therapist may interfere with the patient becoming an active participant in managing her cancer symptoms.

Finally, the therapist appears to assume that this symptom will again be easily treated, which may or may not be the case.

Supporting medical decision-making: For many patients, decisions regarding the initiation, continuation, or cessation of medical treatments are distressing and difficult, particularly with the progression of disease and the failure of first-line treatments. Patients may benefit from exploring the range of feelings that emerge in relation to their treatment choices, as there is often not enough time or space for such reflection to occur in oncology clinics. It is important in such conversations to explore the extent to which a decision to accept or refuse further treatment represents a considered personal decision, a misunderstanding of treatment options or of the risks and benefits, or a decision resulting from perceived pressure from family, loved ones, or healthcare providers. The psychotherapeutic situation may be of particular value in this circumstance by providing an opportunity for patients to explore their thoughts and feelings about treatment, separate from the reactions or concerns of their family, friends, and healthcare team. Neutrality of the therapist with regard to the decisions that patients make about their lives is a time-honored psychotherapeutic position, although this may be more difficult when patients with advanced disease make decisions about their treatment or other aspects of their lives. Patients may intuit the attitudes or views of the therapist, even when they are not explicitly communicated. Rather than attempting to sustain an illusion of neutrality, therapists can sometimes position their attitude about the subject as just one view among the many that might be held about the treatment decision. In some cases, this may be a more realistic position to take than one in which the therapist ostensibly has no opinion whatsoever.

Case Example 2

Benefit from exploring treatment options was evident in a 67-year-old woman with advanced cancer. Her adult son insisted that she pursue further treatment while she eventually came to believe that further treatment would not be effective and would limit her ability to engage in meaningful activities in the time that remained. However, for a long period, she felt internally conflicted about whether to continue to pursue such interventions. She found it difficult to trust her own judgment when further treatment was being proposed by her healthcare providers. She had not found benefit in any of the interventions that she had received, but she wanted to be a "good patient" who was compliant with medical recommendations. She did not want to forego any possibility of prolonging her life, but she also feared that pursuing these options left her little ability to live her life meaningfully. When she discussed this with her son, she found that his focus on further chemotherapy was driven more by his distress than by the literal wish for her to have more systemic treatment. When this was clarified, her son was able to accept his mother's decision not to proceed with treatment and to communicate how much she mattered to him.

Case Example 3

A father of three young children was recently diagnosed with metastatic kidney cancer with a guarded prognosis but was offered chemotherapy by his cancer care team. The patient's father, a surgeon, encouraged him to go ahead with the chemotherapy while the patient's wife, a practitioner in the field of complementary medicine, suggested that he travel to Mexico for a program of vitamin injections instead of chemotherapy.

Patient: "I really feel torn. What would you do in my situation?"

CALM therapeutic responses: Therapists could respond honestly either by saying that they do not know what they would do or by indicating their inclination. However, most important is to encourage the patient to explore his own feeling about the decision, such as by saying "You've told me what your doctors, your father, and your wife think, and you want to know what I think, but it seems most important for us to explore what each of these options means to you. What do you understand about their risks and benefits and what feelings do they evoke?"

The therapeutic strategy is to encourage the patient to reflect on his understanding of the disease and the potential risks and benefits of different treatment options. This may involve helping him to consider the range of feelings he is experiencing related to his treatment decisions and to reach a final decision based on his own balanced view. Personal meanings of these treatment options, which may or may not be in awareness, can also be articulated and understood as one of multiple perspectives that can be entertained on the risks and benefits of these treatment options (e.g., "Accepting chemotherapy means giving in again to my father" or "Refusing the complementary medicine would feel to my wife like a rejection of everything she stands for").

Non-CALM response: "The oncologists wouldn't offer you this chemotherapy if they didn't think it would be helpful. I think for your sake and the sake of your children, you should consider the treatment with more evidence behind it."

Therapists may have greater confidence in established cancer treatments or be more philosophically aligned to the approach being offered by physicians in their own hospital. However, it may be difficult for this young patient—a father, husband, and son—to find his own position because of the high stakes for him and his family and because he is unclear about what he wants. Therapists who align too quickly with the cancer team may complicate matters further. Exploration of the relational dimensions of the patient's decision may allow him to disentangle the multiple and conflicting opinions of others from his own so that he can make a treatment decision that is based on his personal values and priorities, taking the views of everyone into account.

Case Example 4

A woman with metastatic ovarian cancer had begun to develop significant symptoms related to a pleural effusion, requiring more attention to pain and symptom management and indicating progression of her disease. The oncology team had suggested referral to palliative care, which the patient had adamantly refused.

Patient: "I won't agree to palliative care. For me, palliative care means giving up."

CALM therapeutic response: "What did the suggestion of the oncology team to refer you to palliative care mean to you?" and "What is your understanding of what the palliative care team will do?"

The therapeutic strategy is to encourage the patient to reflect upon the personal meaning of the referral to palliative care. Exploring or mentalizing the meaning of this referral and naming and legitimizing her anxieties had a calming effect; it allowed her to reconsider her belief that the referral to palliative care was synonymous with giving up. The therapist was able to explain that patients are referred to the palliative care team for pain and symptom management at different stages of disease and that their active approach to pain and symptom management did not need to be understood as "giving up." Planning for the end of life was reframed as ensuring that her future care would be consistent with her wishes and could co-exist with active approaches to optimizing her quality of life in the present. Eventually, this patient agreed to see the palliative care team and was able to accept symptom control measures and advance care planning without overwhelming anxiety.

Non-CALM responses: "It's up to you. Just let us know if you want to see the palliative care team" or "It's hard for the team to help you if you don't accept their advice."

While this therapist may intend to support the patient's autonomy in decision-making or to encourage her to accept reasonable medical advice, these approaches may close off emotional exploration and limit the opportunity to process the fears generated by the proposed referral to palliative care.

Developing collaborative relationships with healthcare providers: The relationship of the patient with the treating physician or oncologist is often profoundly important to the patient as a source of information, guidance, and support. The perceived fallibility of healthcare providers, the lapses in the continuity of care that may occur, and the limitations in healthcare resources may be threatening to patients and their families. Such perceived disruptions may trigger attachment-related fears of dependency, burden, rejection, or abandonment. Patients may respond to this by withdrawal, by intensified help-seeking, or with the contradictory posture of being both help-seeking and help-rejecting, which may further complicate relations with the healthcare team. Empathic understanding of the patient's experience may support or repair the alliance with the treatment team when it has been disrupted. Therapists in this situation must work to maintain a balanced perspective and be prepared to act as an advocate or mediator between the patient and other caregivers.

Case Example 5

A man with recently diagnosed metastatic pharyngeal cancer from a rural community described himself as highly independent and previously very healthy with little experience as a patient. He had been prescribed an aggressive combination of chemotherapy and radiation therapy that would require him to move away from his family farm to the city for several weeks of daily treatment.

Patient: "I feel this hospital operates like a big conveyor belt and I need to just shut up and get on it or not come back."

CALM therapeutic response: "It sounds like you have been experiencing this place as an unfeeling machine. How would you like to be treated?"

The therapeutic strategy is to help this patient understand his own experiences and expectations in relation to the medical team and consider practical solutions to his dilemma. His feelings about the impersonal nature of medical care were validated and understood in terms of overarching feelings about life in a big city and the loss of human values in this setting. The therapist validated his reactions to the inevitable loss of individuality that may occur in a large treatment center and explored alternative approaches to address the potential isolation from his family. His subsequent communication with the medical team about his experience reassured him about their interest in him as a person and facilitated a practical solution to his concerns, which involved assistance with transportation to and from the farm during his chemotherapy.

Non-CALM response: "I'm sure your medical team really cares about you."

While the therapist may intend to reassure the patient with this statement, it may be experienced by the patient as dismissive and does not facilitate mentalization or reflection on his experience or assumptions about the reactions of others. Finally, it does not support the patient in developing a more collaborative approach to his care, which may allow him to revise his initial assumptions.

DOMAIN 2: CHANGES IN SELF AND RELATIONS WITH CLOSE OTHERS

The general goals of this domain are to:

1. Empathically explore the patient's experience in relationships with close friends and family in the context of advanced disease;
2. Facilitate understanding of the impact of the disease and treatment on the patient's self-concept and relationships with close others;
3. Explore anxieties and conflicts about dependency and caregiving and barriers to accepting support in the face of progressive disease; and
4. Conduct joint sessions with the primary caregiver, when feasible, to explore relational dynamics and support the couple in anticipating and preparing for future difficulties. This may include attention to the needs and experience of children and other family members.

Suggested probes to initiate discussion (with patient and/or caregiver):

- "Tell me what you are like in relationships? What concerns do you tend to have?"
- If more specificity is needed, "Do you tend to be self-reliant or to be someone who is able to lean on others in times of stress?"
- "Have you found that cancer has changed the way people behave towards you?" and if so, "How?"
- "How do you want others to treat you now that you are ill?"
- "How has your cancer affected your partner (or other primary caregiver)?"
- "How has your cancer affected your children?"
- "What has changed in your household since the cancer?"
- "Do you talk about your cancer at home?" and if so, "What do you discuss? What don't you discuss? Is this working?"

Receiving and providing needed care and support: The experience of advanced disease often leads to dramatic changes in the household division of labor, financial responsibilities, parenting roles, and emotional and physical intimacy. Many patients with advanced disease can flexibly seek and obtain the emotional and practical support that they want and need from their loved ones. In some cases, however, attachment fears interfere with the ability to seek or obtain support from caregivers and may trigger responses from them that are unwanted or disturbing. Identifying and acknowledging the attachment needs of patients and their caregivers and the adjustments that may be required from both may help to restore equilibrium and mutual support in these relationships. The failure to resolve relational concerns and disruptions may enhance the patient's sense of isolation and trigger the onset or exacerbation of depressive symptoms.

Case Example 1

A woman with metastatic lung cancer was midway through a course of chemotherapy. She tended to be fearful that she will be unsupported or abandoned, reflecting her anxious attachment style. She repeatedly called her oncology team with questions and requests for more frequent appointments. The team was feeling increasingly frustrated by this patient's demands and her inability to calm herself despite frequent and repeated reassurance.

Patient: "I don't think I can make it through the rest of my chemotherapy. I really think I'm going to need way more than just six sessions with you."

CALM therapeutic response: "I've noticed that you often doubt your ability to cope. What makes you feel you will be unable to cope?" Then, "I see that you have made it through half your chemotherapy. What has worked so far to help you get to this point?"

The therapeutic strategy is one of empathic understanding of this patient's feelings of need and exploration of her anxieties about abandonment. There is also an attempt to identify this patient's adaptive strengths and thereby build her confidence in her own coping and support system.

Non-CALM responses: "CALM therapy only allows for six sessions so you'll have to make use of me in the time we have left" or "Don't worry, I can make an exception, and we can schedule as many CALM sessions as you need."

The therapist may be trying to set realistic limits in terms of the care that can be provided or to reassure this patient with promises of unlimited support. However, these approaches treat as fact this patient's assumption that she will not be able to cope in the future. They do not support reflection on her tendency to experience intense need in the face of difficulties and her lack of confidence in her own internal resources.

Case Example 2

A man with metastatic prostate cancer had been referred to palliative care due to recent physical decline. He had an avoidant attachment style characterized by inflexible self-reliance and minimization of distress. The palliative care team had been concerned about his recent depressive symptoms, social withdrawal, and feelings of hopelessness and encouraged him to seek psychotherapeutic support.

Patient: "I really wasn't sure about coming for psychotherapy. How could talking about it make any difference in my situation?"

CALM therapeutic response: "Talking may not change your disease, but have you ever found that communicating what you feel has been helpful?" Then, "Have you found 'going it alone' to be getting more difficult as your disease has progressed? Can you imagine that talking with me about your situation might help with your feelings of sadness and isolation?"

The therapeutic strategy is one of curiosity, exploring doubts and hopes about emotional communication and support. Paradoxically, the exploration of doubts and fears about the expression of feelings may mark the beginning of a meaningful engagement. This may also lead to exploration of other relational patterns in the patient's life and of obstacles to obtaining appropriate support. The nonintrusive and implicit offer of support does not imply weakness or a complete loss of independence and may help reverse the patient's defensive withdrawal and the cascade of consequences that has led to his depressive symptoms. The subsequent renegotiation of the patient's attachment relationships may allow him to be better able to accept support, to retain some sense of his own autonomy, and to be less likely to see strength and weakness as dichotomous attributes.

Non-CALM response: "Yes, it's true, words can't change what is happening to you" or "You can't keep it all bottled up inside. Talking about your feelings may provide relief."

With the first response, the therapist may be attempting to empathize with this patient's experience and not exaggerate the benefits that a brief psychotherapy can provide, but it treats as fact this patient's assumption that sharing an experience cannot provide any relief. The second response contrasts with the first by expressing the therapist's belief in the potential benefits of the psychotherapeutic relationship but does not allow exploration of this patient's individual concerns and hesitance.

Case Example 3

A woman with metastatic cervical cancer had recently completed a course of chemotherapy. She had an anxious attachment style, with an intensely expressed need for support from others and a fear that it will not be available. Following a recent computed tomography (CT) scan that showed disease progression and then two missed scheduled CALM sessions, she came to a CALM session several weeks later.

Patient: "I've been feeling so overwhelmed. No one is helping me."

CALM therapeutic response: "When you received those upsetting CT results, you cancelled a few of our sessions. What stopped you from coming to our sessions then?"

The therapeutic strategy is to acknowledge the patient's distress and to explore her paradoxical relational tendency to withdraw from relationships while simultaneously experiencing an intense need for support.

Non-CALM response: "If you don't come to regularly scheduled CALM sessions, how can I be of help to you?"

While the therapist may be trying to encourage the patient to engage in the therapy, this statement does not empathize with the patient's experience and might be interpreted as critical or rejecting and actually decrease the likelihood that she would come to the therapist when distressed in the future.

Working with caregivers in CALM: An integral aspect of CALM is the invitation to the patient-identified primary caregiver to attend one or more CALM sessions. It is emphasized to the patient that this is a routine aspect of CALM, although patients can decide whether they want to invite a caregiver and when. The goal of CALM joint sessions is to provide another viewpoint on the patient and caregiver's individual and shared perspectives and to bolster cohesion and support in the relational unit. The approach in joint sessions includes exploration of the relationship history and the shared management of past crises, encouragement of empathic understanding and mentalizing the other (i.e., "What do you think your husband/wife is feeling or thinking?"), and acknowledgment of the shared and nonshared experience. The aim of these joint sessions is to facilitate greater mutual attunement and to assist in repairing disruptions in the attachment relationship triggered by the illness. Patients and caregivers may be encouraged to make small adjustments and consider new care-seeking or caregiving behaviors that may increase the sense of felt support within the relationship.

Case Example 4

A couple married for 10 years had long had independence in their lives and careers despite mutual shared interests. When the patient's metastatic melanoma led to his need for more emotional support, his partner arranged for him to be referred for individual psychosocial support.

Patient: "I don't think I need this. I'm really worried mostly about my wife. I think she is the one who needs to see a therapist. Could you talk with her?"

CALM therapeutic response: "What makes you worried about her? What do you imagine she is thinking and feeling?" And then, "It's interesting that each of you is worried about the other. Would you be open to inviting her to our next session to talk together about how you are coping as a family?"

The therapeutic strategy is to encourage empathic consideration of what his wife may be feeling and to reframe the cancer as a shared problem, although one with different challenges for each of them. By seeing them together, there is the possibility that greater attunement and support could be obtained within the relationship that will benefit them both long after CALM therapy is complete.

Supporting children and other family members: A common problem for patients and caregivers is what to tell children and other family members about the illness, when to tell them, and how to support them throughout the illness process. In some cases, fears of dying and death may lead to avoidance of discussions about the illness, while in other cases fears may lead to frightening rumination on the topic. The CALM approach is not prescriptive about how, when, or whether prognostic information should be communicated within the family, although the more visible the effects of the disease and treatment become, the more there may be need for discussion about it. Such discussions with children and other family members can begin with enquiry about what they do understand about the patient's condition and what they would like to know. Patients may also benefit from the reminder that discussions about this are usually best viewed as a process, rather than as a single event. Reflection within CALM sessions involves consideration of the perspectives and needs of children and other family members and the fears and worries about what would happen if there was more open communication. When these conversations do happen, parents can be encouraged to be attuned to the reaction of the child or family member, to maintain a flexible stance and willingness to talk when the child or family member is ready, and to communicate that support will be available.

Case Example 5

A married man with metastatic colon cancer had a six-year-old son. He and his wife told his son about the cancer at the time of his original diagnosis and surgery but not about the cancer recurrence or chemotherapy.

Patient: "I can't help thinking 'What's the point?' He'll eventually have to deal with it, but I don't see the reason for frightening him now."

CALM therapeutic response: "What do you believe that your son thinks is wrong with you?" and "What are you afraid would happen if you did tell him about the recurrence?"

The therapeutic strategy is to encourage reflection on the reasons behind the parents' decision not to tell their son and to help them distinguish between their own emotions and those of their child. Helping these parents manage their own anxieties about the discussion with their son may be a necessary first step before helpful communication with their son can take place. This discussion can begin by enquiring about their son's understanding of the situation and what he might like more information about.

Non-CALM response: "Children often know more than you think. You need to talk to your child openly about what's happening to you to help him cope with his feelings."

While the therapist may believe that open communication about cancer within families is in the best interest of the child, this directive approach does not allow for an understanding of the parents' concerns about open communication to emerge, nor does it facilitate their finding an approach that fits with their own values, preferences, and concerns.

DOMAIN 3: SPIRITUALITY AND THE SENSE OF MEANING AND PURPOSE

The general goals of this module are to:

1. Empathically explore the patient's spiritual or religious beliefs and current sources of meaning and purpose in life;
2. Help the patient make sense of the experience of their disease based on their life experiences, personality, and the nature and course of their disease and symptoms;

3. Support a narrative review that helps the patient identify the perceived accomplishments, legacies, regrets, and disappointments of their life; and
4. Help the patient to reflect on and reconsider their priorities and goals in the face of a shortened life span.

Suggested probes to initiate discussion:
Questions of meaning and purpose are embedded within almost all dimensions of advanced disease but may sometimes require specific exploration for them to be addressed. These issues may be least likely to be raised by patients in CALM and may not be addressed without explicit prompts or inquiry. Some specific probes include:

- "How do you make sense of what is happening to you?"
- "What has been important to you in life?" "What are you most proud of? Have there been disappointments or regrets?"
- "How have your priorities or values changed since you became ill?"
- "What do you feel gives your life most meaning?" or "What do you rely on most for support?"
- "Is spirituality or religion important in your life?" and if so, "What does it mean for you now?"

Understanding the personal meaning of suffering and dying: Meaning-making is an adaptive response of humans to help manage what is frightening and seems uncontrollable. This may help to explain why spirituality and the sense of meaning and purpose become important for many individuals near the end of life (LeMay & Wilson, 2008). For some, the crisis of illness and dying leads to a strengthening of long-held religious or philosophical views. For others, it raises painful struggles with such questions as "Why me?" "What comes next?" and "Why must my family suffer?" One patient with advanced cancer who had lived a virtuous life said, "God has some explaining, some serious explaining, to do." Another pleaded with God not to punish her by causing her disease to progress. By exploring how patients make sense of their situation, therapists can facilitate and support meaning-making as an adaptive way to cope with a situation beyond their control.

Case Example 1

A woman with metastatic breast cancer had withdrawn recently from a support group for women with breast cancer.

Patient: "If I hear one more story about how cancer has been a blessing in disguise, I'll scream."

CALM therapeutic response: "The cancer experience is highly individual. How have you found that cancer has affected your outlook on life?"

The therapeutic strategy is to help this patient create her own narrative about the cancer and its meaning for her, including the possibility of multiple personal experiences and perspectives, rather than to either encourage a more positive outlook or validate her negative one.

Non-CALM response: "Yes, cancer is a terrible disease. It's awful that we can't acknowledge that and talk about it in support groups."

While this therapist may intend to empathize with the patient and validate her experience, this response prevents reflection on the multiple possible meanings of cancer.

Evaluating priorities and goals in the face of advanced disease: As the illness progresses, previously important goals and activities, particularly those related to physicality or productivity, may no longer be achievable or meaningful (Yalom, 1980). The perceived shortness of time raises questions about how to spend the time remaining, which may require a reconsideration of life priorities and goals. Helping patients to live more meaningfully in the present can alleviate and may even prevent the demoralization that can be a complication of disease progression.

Case Example 2

A man with three young children and a diagnosis of metastatic esophageal cancer described a long history of feeling torn between the demands of his family and his dreams of devoting himself more fully to his love of music composition. This conflict led to a feeling of dissatisfaction and of "failing on all fronts." He was told that his disease had progressed and while the oncology team was clear that his treatment was not curative, they were encouraged by his premorbid good health and told him that he may have several years of good quality of life with chemotherapy.

Patient: "I guess that's the final 'nail in the coffin' of my music career. And my kids, well . . . all I can see is my empty chair at the dinner table."

CALM therapeutic response: "I understand that you feel all is lost now and that all of your dreams have not been fulfilled." And later, after exploration of these feelings, "If you do have a limited amount of healthy time left, how can you imagine spending it?"

The therapeutic strategy is first to acknowledge the grief felt in the face of perceived losses, which included unfulfilled dreams of being the "perfect" father and a prolific musician. Then, by initiating reflection on new priorities and goals, the therapist creates space in which the patient may begin to plan to live meaningfully in the face of a shortened life span. The patient subsequently expressed a renewed commitment to fatherhood and to spending time with his children and began to feel that his cancer gave him license to focus some of his spare time on his music. The result was both renewed engagement with his family and a prolific period of creativity, all while undergoing chemotherapy.

Non-CALM response: "We all have to face these limits. This is the human condition. Being a husband and father are both meaningful accomplishments though."

While the therapist may intend to join with the patient regarding the reality of death as a finite end, this statement does not validate his patient's expression of grief. In addition, it preempts the patient's own reflection on goals and presupposes that commitment and dedication to family should be experienced as meaningful.

DOMAIN 4: PREPARING FOR THE FUTURE, HOPE, AND MORTALITY

The general goals of this module are to:

1. Empathically explore the patients' attitudes towards the future and their hopes and fears about living with and dying from advanced disease;
2. Support and encourage acknowledgment of anticipatory fears and anxieties and help to maintain the balance of living and dying; and
3. Attend to advance care planning, life closure, and death preparation.

Suggested probes to initiate discussion:

- "When you look to the future, what do you see ahead of you?"
- "Do you think about dying and death?" and if so, "What do you think about?" If there is distress associated with thoughts of dying and death, "What are your biggest fears about dying or death?"
- "What might help you prepare for what lies ahead?"

Acknowledgment of anticipatory fears: The power of "positive thinking" to cure or slow the progression of disease is frequently touted to cancer patients by their community, the media, and even the healthcare establishment, although the weight of scientific evidence does not support this view (Garssen, 2004; Goodwin et al., 2001). Exclusively positive thinking can almost never be sustained in the context of progression of advanced disease. Hope in such individuals is most secure when it is not based on false expectations that are likely to be shattered. As the disease progresses and symptoms and disability increase, avoidant strategies become less tenable. Pressure from family, friends, or healthcare providers to "think positively" may have the effect of silencing or dismissing patients' and caregivers' fears, leaving them feeling isolated. For many patients, the opportunity in CALM to speak openly of dying and death, with normalization of their fears, can be profoundly validating and calming.

Case Example 1

A woman with lymphoma now had recurrent disease after stem cell transplant and was receiving palliative radiation therapy.

Patient: "What frightens me most now is dying a bad death."

CALM therapeutic response: "What would a 'bad death' look like for you?" And later, after exploration of her fears, "What could you do now to try to avoid that kind of death?"

The therapeutic strategy is to understand with this patient what frightens her when she thinks about dying and death. The therapist demonstrates a willingness to reflect on a topic that may not be comfortably explored alone or with family due to the terror it generates in the patient or in others. The therapist then shifts to help her consider strategies to achieve a "good death" or "good enough death." This may generate a greater sense of control and lead to calming of the patient and may initiate practical discussions around advance care planning and death preparation.

Balance of living and dying: A common dilemma for caregivers of those with advanced disease is whether and when to challenge or explore patients' so-called denial of illness (Rodin & Zimmermann, 2008). In some cases, what has been regarded as denial of illness actually represents a heightened importance of living in the present, stemming from an exquisite awareness of the prognosis, rather than from denial of it. In other cases, the unwillingness to think about the stage of disease or the severity of symptoms may manifest in delayed help-seeking or as a lack of planning for disease progression and the end of life. Although denial and avoidance may have adaptive functions, their meaning and consequences should be explored when they interfere with appropriate treatment or necessary personal tasks, such as arranging a will or settling personal financial matters. In other cases, death preoccupation may interfere with the capacity to sustain meaningful engagement in life. An important goal of CALM is to help patients with advanced and life-threatening disease sustain the balance of living and dying. Such "double awareness" allows them to plan, mourn their losses, and continue to live life in the present.

Case Example 2

A woman with metastatic stomach cancer was seen with her husband for one session. They both understood that her treatment was not curative, but they did not discuss her advancing disease or the possibility of her death. At this joint session, the husband expressed anger with the oncologist for mentioning prognosis and advance care planning to his wife at her last appointment, although the physician also proposed that she consider participating in a clinical trial.

Husband: "I can't believe that she would bring this up with her. It is so damaging to patients when physicians take away all of their hope. We're going to fight this."

CALM therapeutic response: "Was what the oncologist said a surprise to you?" And then, "It sounds like you feel you need to choose between planning for disease progression or active treatment. Is it possible to do both at the same time?"

The therapeutic strategy is to introduce the possibility that the couple might find a way to both fight the disease and face the possibility of her death. The ongoing capacity to sustain this duality may, in fact, be the central feature that allows many individuals to face the end without resignation, retreat, or the narrowing of experience.

Non-CALM response: "I know you both understand that this cancer is not curable. At some point don't you have to discuss what lies ahead and prepare?"

While the therapist may believe that open acknowledgment and acceptance of death is a healthy approach to the end of life, this perspective is not shared by the patient and her husband at this time. Further, encouraging the patient either to "fight" or to "accept" the disease progression ignores the potential duality of engaging in life while also facing death, a capacity which we have termed "double awareness" (Rodin & Zimmermann, 2008).

Advance care planning, life closure, and death preparation: Research with patients and families on the concept of a good death has consistently identified advance care planning, life closure, and death preparation activities as important components of a positive dying experience (Hales et al., 2008). These may include making end-of-life care wishes explicit, planning funeral and financial arrangements, saying goodbye to family and friends, or working on "legacy projects" such as letters, videos, or gifts for loved ones. Creating opportunities to reflect on these issues, without a requirement to do so, may allow patients to experience a sense of closure and control and to feel as though they are leaving a positive legacy behind them. Such intervention may also significantly benefit family and friends who will survive them.

Case Example 3

A woman with metastatic colon cancer had a long-standing history of mild anxiety, which she typically managed by gathering information and preparing in advance for potentially difficult problems. Although her disease was stable on chemotherapy, she asked her oncologist for information about end-of-life care at her previous appointment.

Patient response: "My oncologist didn't want to talk about it and told me I don't need to worry about this yet."

CALM therapeutic response: "What kind of information were you looking for? What do you think you need to do to prepare for the possibility of dying?"

The therapeutic strategy is to validate and normalize the patient's wishes to attend to life closure and death preparation, even though death is not imminent. Such adaptive death preparation should be distinguished from a morbid preoccupation with dying and death that impairs quality of life or psychosocial functioning.

Non-CALM response: "She's right, you're not dying right now. Maybe this is a time to focus on living."

While the therapist may mean to allay her anxiety, this response dismisses a coping strategy that is adaptive for this patient.

CONCLUSION

The four domains of CALM provide a framework for clinicians to ensure that patients are given the opportunity to explore the range of issues that commonly emerge over the course of advanced cancer. Asking open-ended questions is often all that is required for patients' concerns to emerge, even in the most emotionally sensitive areas, such as mortality and meaning in life. For those facing mortality the perceived shortness of time may contribute to the depth and intimacy of the therapeutic relationship even within a brief psychotherapy intervention. The CALM domains are often interrelated and exploration of one domain frequently leads to implicit or explicit exploration of other domains. The art of CALM involves addressing the CALM domains in the sequence and depth that are desired by the patient, with simultaneous attention to the therapeutic relationship, affect regulation, and attachment security.

REFERENCES

Garssen, B. (2004). Psychological factors and cancer development: Evidence after 30 years of research. *Clinical Psychology Review, 24*(3), 315–338.

Goodwin, P. J., Leszcz, M., Ennis, M., Koopmans, J., Vincent, L., Guther, H., Drysdale, E., Hundleby, M., Chochinov, H. M., Navarro, M., Speca, M., Masterson, J., Dohan, L., Sela, R., Warren, B., Paterson, A., Pritchard, K. I., Arnold, A., Doll, R., O'Reilly, S. E., Quirt, G., Hood, N., & Hunter, J. (2001). The effect of group psychosocial support on survival in metastatic breast cancer. *The New England Journal of Medicine, 345*(24), 1719–1726.

Hales, S., Zimmermann, C., & Rodin, G. (2008). The quality of dying and death. *Archives of Internal Medicine, 168*(9), 912–918.

LeMay, K., & Wilson, K. G. (2008). Treatment of existential distress in life threatening illness: A review of manualized interventions. *Clinical Psychology Review, 28*(3), 472–493.

Rodin, G., & Zimmermann, C. (2008). Psychoanalytic reflections on mortality: A reconsideration. *Journal of the American Academy of Psychoanalysis and Dynamic Psychiatry, 36*(1), 181–196.

Yalom, I. D. (1980). *Existential psychotherapy*. Basic Books.

CHAPTER 16

Utilizing Measures in Clinical Practice and Supervision

INTRODUCTION

We have paid meticulous attention to the development, validation, and utilization of self-report measures as part of our research program (see Chapter 10 of this volume). However, we soon discovered that these measures are also extremely useful clinical tools for therapists and for those monitoring the course of the therapy. The following text outlines the use of relevant psychometric measures in Managing Cancer and Living Meaningful (CALM) clinical practice and supervision and discusses the format and benefit of ongoing peer supervision in CALM.

THE USE OF MEASURES WITHIN CALM THERAPY

Self-report measures are routinely completed by patients at the onset of CALM therapy and after three and six months to guide the therapist regarding CALM content, process, and outcome, and to inform CALM supervision. These measures are:

1. The Death and Dying Distress Scale (DADDS) (Lo, Hales, et al., 2011; Shapiro et al., 2020) is a validated 15-item scale measuring death anxiety in patients with advanced cancer. Unlike other death anxiety measures (Neimeyer, 1994), the DADDS is designed for populations facing

imminent death. It addresses fears about the dying process and distress about lost opportunities and self-perceived burden placed on others as a result of impending mortality (see Appendix A).

2. The modified and brief Experiences in Close Relationships scale (ECR-M16; Lo et al., 2009) is now a widely used 16-item measure of attachment security, which has demonstrated reliability and validity. It provides subscale scores assessing attachment anxiety and avoidance (see Appendix B).

3. The Quality of Life at the End of Life-Cancer Scale (QUAL-EC; Lo, Burman, et al., 2011) assesses quality of life in patients near the end of life and includes four subscales, which are:

   a. *Symptom control*, which measures the frequency, severity, and interference caused by physical symptoms of cancer experienced in the previous month;

   b. *Preparation for the end of life*, which assesses the extent to which the patient is worried about impending issues, such as financial strain, death and dying, and family members' ability to cope;

   c. *Relationship with healthcare providers*, which assesses the extent to which patients feel informed and able to participate in decisions about their care; and

   d. *Life completion*, which measures the extent to which patients feel connected to others and feel a sense of meaning and peace (see Appendix C).

4. The Patient Health Questionnaire-9 (PHQ-9; Kroenke et al., 2001) is a reliable and valid 9-item measure of depression that has been used widely with advanced cancer patients (e.g., Ell et al., 2008). We added one additional item assessing intent to cause self-harm (item 9a: "Is there a chance you would do something to end your life?"), which has been part of routine distress screening at our cancer center (Li et al., 2016; see Appendix D).

In many cases, the patient's scores on psychometric scales mirror the therapist's clinical observations, providing a more precise quantification of important aspects of the patient experience. The measure of attachment security, for instance, sheds light on the relational difficulties of patients and can inform the therapeutic posture of the therapist in relation to the patient (Tan et al., 2005). In some cases, there are discrepancies between the content of the sessions and the patient's scores on the measures. These discrepancies may occur when patients are more comfortable reporting their distress on a psychometric measure than to the therapist or when distress is not adequately explored in session by the therapist. In these instances, the patient's scores provide a quantitative indication of distress that cannot easily be obtained in the CALM sessions. Finally, when patients complete measures before, during, and at the end of therapy, this provides an additional lens on the effect of therapy. When patients are seen for several sessions and their distress scores remain high, modifications to the therapeutic approach may be indicated. Bringing the measures into therapy can also provide an opportunity for the patient and therapist to discuss progress in therapy and adjust the content or process as needed. This process is in keeping with the recognition, across different psychotherapeutic modalities, that routine outcome monitoring and feedback enhances psychotherapeutic care provision (Lambert, 2010).

Therapists in our center receive a one-page report of calculated measure scores that can provide a picture at a glance of their patient's profile. This report also marks the cut-off points for moderate and high scores based on our previous research. The CALM research program has also relied upon the CALM Treatment Integrity Measure (CTIM; see Appendix E) and the Clinical Evaluation Questionnaire (CEQ; see Appendix F) to ensure, respectively, the integrity of the intervention and the cumulative perceived benefit of the intervention from the perspective of the patient (see Chapter 10 of this volume). We are now beginning to incorporate the use of both the CTIM and the CEQ into our clinical practice and training.

CALM SUPERVISION

A significant and integral aspect of the CALM approach is ongoing peer supervision that begins during training and continues on an ongoing basis for experienced CALM therapists. These group meetings not only help to ensure treatment integrity but also foster ongoing CALM skill development and may help clinicians manage their own existential distress. Supervision provides a forum for ongoing therapist development, collegial support, and fostering of realistic expectations. It may also mitigate against burnout by providing guidance, support, the setting of realistic expectations, and reflective space (Maslach et al., 1996; Pessin et al., 2015; see Chapter 11 of this volume).

CALM supervision groups ideally contain no more than 8 to 10 therapists with a mix of training and experience levels. The intended model, once basic skills have developed, is peer supervision with all encouraged to take part in considering how to support the therapist in delivering CALM to the patient under discussion. Given that therapist disclosure about countertransference and therapeutic challenges is encouraged, assurance about the confidentiality of the discussions is essential.

Therapists are invited to present new or in-progress cases, and there is an ongoing rotating schedule of planned case discussions. Initially, the therapist presents a summary of the patient; the reason for referral; their current distress levels; content relating to the four CALM domains; process issues related to attachment style, affect regulation, and mentalizing ability; death-related distress; reference to transference/countertransference issues and the therapeutic relationship; and the therapist's overall impression and approach to future treatment (see Appendixes G and H). More experienced therapists may choose to focus the discussion on a particular question or challenge they are facing. Patient measure scores are reviewed, and, if available, an audiotape or videotape segment selected by the therapist may be presented. The group may help to further formulate an understanding of the patient and provide suggestions for therapeutic interventions and goals. Therapists are encouraged to present cases more than once to consider the success and effect of prior suggestions and to review outcomes.

For the past decade, we have held an ongoing weekly multidisciplinary CALM supervision group at the Princess Margaret Cancer Centre that includes new and more experienced CALM therapists. It has served as an important tool for development and refinement of the intervention. Over time, we have found that there are several important ingredients of an effective CALM supervision group, which include a culture of safety and participation where therapists are invited to reflect on perceived missteps, failures, uncertainties, and ambivalence; emphasis on CALM-specific aspects of therapy and how the approach is different from other brief therapies; and frequent modeling of the therapy with sharing of videos and audiotapes.

Over the years, some themes have repeatedly emerged in supervision. Many of these highlight the tensions inherent in this type of work. Common therapist challenges include:

- Introducing painful topics while supporting and respecting the patient's defenses;
- Overcoming feelings of uselessness and futility in order to engage helpfully with the patient;
- Knowledge of the disease course of common cancers which patients may not want to or be ready to discuss;
- Supporting the sometimes conflicting needs of both patients and caregivers;
- Facilitating change while recognizing unresolvable disappointments; and

- Ending therapy with the knowledge that more adversity or problems may lie ahead for the patient and their family as the cancer advances.

Regular online international supervisory meetings in diverse regions have been conducted to support training and research as part of our Global CALM program. These meetings have been essential to support expertise in the delivery of CALM throughout the world and to understand regional and cultural differences in such issues as the expression of distress, emotional intimacy, attachment relationships, the role of family and community, and the value placed on autonomy and individual accomplishment. The learning process in these supervision groups has been reciprocal, with the feedback and experience of global CALM therapists and trainees informing the refinement of CALM in an iterative fashion. Although the cultural relevance and acceptability of CALM has been demonstrated in diverse global settings, its semi-structured nature allows local therapists to deliver it in their own voice and decide, based on their own judgment, the cultural relevance and appropriateness of specific CALM elements for their patients.

CONCLUSION

The CALM project has integrated clinical care with research and education from its inception. The development and application of relevant, psychometrically valid measurement tools to guide clinical care and monitor therapeutic outcomes has helped to refine the CALM intervention. The process of supervision has also helped to create a community of CALM clinicians who learn from each other and provide mutual support in facing the ongoing challenges of helping patients and their families live with advanced disease.

REFERENCES

Ell, K., Xie, B., Quon, B., Quinn, D. I., Dwight-Johnson, M., & Lee, P. J. (2008). Randomized controlled trial of collaborative care management of depression among low-income patients with cancer. *Journal of Clinical Oncology, 26*(27), 4488–4496.

Kroenke, K., Spitzer, R. L., & Williams, J. B. (2001). The PHQ-9: Validity of a brief depression severity measure. *Journal of General Internal Medicine, 16*(9), 606–613.

Lambert, M. J. (2010). *Prevention of treatment failure: The use of measuring, monitoring and feedback in clinical practice.* American Psychological Association.

Li, M., Macedo, A., Crawford, S., Bagha, S., Leung, Y. W., Zimmermann, C., Fitzgerald, B., Wyatt, M., Stuart-McEwan, T., & Rodin, G. (2016). Easier said than done: Keys to successful implementation of the Distress Assessment and Response Tool (DART) program. *Journal of Oncology Practice, 12*(5), e513–e526. doi: 10.1200/JOP.2015.010066.

Lo, C., Burman, D., Swami, N., Gagliese, L., Rodin, G., & Zimmermann, C. (2011). Validation of the QUAL-EC for assessing quality of life in patients with advanced cancer. *European Journal of Cancer, 47*(4), 554–560.

Lo, C., Hales, S., Zimmermann, C., Gagliese, L., Rydall, A., & Rodin, G. (2011). Measuring death-related anxiety in advanced cancer: Preliminary psychometrics of the Death and Dying Distress Scale. *Journal of Pediatric Hematology/Oncology, 33* (Suppl 2), S140–S145.

Lo, C., Walsh, A., Mikulincer, M., Gagliese, L., Zimmermann, C., & Rodin, G. (2009). Measuring attachment security in patients with advanced cancer: Psychometric properties of a modified and brief Experiences in Close Relationships scale. *Psycho-Oncology, 18*(5), 490–499.

Maslach, C., Jackson, S. E., & Leiter, M. P. (1996). *Maslach Burnout Inventory Manual* (3rd edition). Consulting Psychologists Press.

Neimeyer, R. A. (Ed.). (1994). *Death anxiety handbook: Research, instrumentation, and application*. Taylor & Francis.

Pessin, H., Fenn, N., Hendriksen, E., DeRosa, A. P., & Applebaum, A. (2015). Existential distress among healthcare providers caring for patients at the end of life. *Current Opinion in Supportive and Palliative Care, 9*(1), 77–86.

Shapiro, G. K., Mah, K., Li, M., Zimmermann, C., Hales, S., & Rodin, G. (2020). Validation of the Death and Dying Distress Scale in patients with advanced cancer. *Psycho-Oncology.* 2020 Dec 26. doi: 10.1002/pon.5620. Epub ahead of print.

Tan, A., Zimmermann, C., & Rodin, G. (2005). Interpersonal processes in palliative care: An attachment perspective on the patient-clinician relationship. *Palliative Medicine, 19*(2), 143–150.

CHAPTER 17

CALM Therapy Cases

INTRODUCTION

The following text presents case summaries based on actual patients treated with Managing Cancer and Living Meaningful (CALM) in our setting (identifying details have been changed to maintain confidentiality). These summaries illustrate how the process and content of CALM unfold in the treatment of specific patients.

CASE SUMMARY: THE PROFESSOR

Ms. M was a 66-year-old woman, originally from Argentina, who had immigrated to Canada in early adulthood. She was a former professor of biology who had never married and, as a single parent, had raised a son who was now in his 30s. Ms. M had been diagnosed with endometrial cancer five years earlier and had received numerous chemotherapies and participated in several clinical trials. However, her disease relentlessly metastasized to her lymph nodes, lung, and liver. When she was withdrawn from a phase I clinical trial due to internal bleeding from peritoneal metastases, Ms. M became intensely distressed and felt a sense of great urgency to start another trial as soon as possible. She was referred for CALM after another patient on the same clinical trial suggested it might be helpful.

The Initial Session: A "Horrifying Vision"

Ms. M described herself in the first session as "stalwart" and not a "weak" person who would be prone to depression or anxiety. However, being unable to be physically active, to care for her aging parents, or to continue with her academic work made her feel that she was "of no use" and that her life had no meaning. She equated being taken off cancer treatment with "doing nothing," which meant, to her, that she "might as well be dying." Her predominant affect in the first session was anger directed toward herself, her disease, and the clinical trial team. When the therapist commented on this, Ms. M said that she had indeed been angry since she was removed from the clinical trial. However, what emerged from this discussion was that Ms. M felt empowered by her anger and struggled more with underlying feelings of helplessness and vulnerability that she had been trying hard to keep out of awareness. When the therapist asked what it was that she might be trying not to think and feel, Ms. M described a "horrifying vision" of a scene in which she was lying in a hospital bed, frail and thin, with her adult son sitting beside her, a witness to her deterioration. This picture filled her with terror, and she imagined it would be similarly intolerable for her son.

Ms. M's view of herself and her situation, and her unrecognized affect state, could be understood in light of her avoidant attachment style. Her self-reliance had been highly adaptive and had served her well as a single parent and throughout her career in a competitive academic field. However, her fear of vulnerability and her belief that dependency on others reflected weakness were distressing and influenced her treatment decision-making, driving her toward ever more debilitating clinical trials. Her need to be self-sufficient prevented her from accessing emotional support from family and friends, which could have helped her cope with her growing anger and fear.

The Middle Sessions: Redefining Courage

Over the course of Ms. M's nine-session therapy, the therapist continued to attend to her unacknowledged affect, to support mentalization, and to encourage renegotiation of attachment relationships. This involved acknowledging Ms. M's independent and active approach to life as a strength, while also considering alternative views about the burden that she believed her dependence might impose on others. Ms. M and her son began to engage in more open communication about her cancer. As Ms. M began to decline physically, she came to find her son's involvement in the management of her illness to be more tolerable and meaningful. The therapist also questioned her belief that palliative care meant being "passive" and "doing nothing," suggesting instead that advance care planning might require the same active determination and courage she had brought to participation in each new clinical trial.

The Final Session: The Image in Reality

Ms. M was not able to engage in another clinical trial, although she remained hopeful of this until her final admission to the hospital with a respiratory infection. At that time, her strength and mobility were declining, and she agreed to a palliative care consultation for symptom management. The therapist was able to visit Ms. M in her hospital room just days before her death and found her lying in bed, smiling, with her son at her side holding her hand. Ms. M felt comforted by the presence of her son at the end of life, a stark contrast to the horrific image that she had recounted at the start of CALM.

CASE SUMMARY: FINDING A HOME

Ms. A was a 65-year-old married woman with ovarian cancer who was randomized to receive CALM as part of the large CALM trial. She had participated in numerous other clinical trials, but her disease had been refractory to all of them. She felt close to her three adult children who wanted her to continue pursuing further clinical trials because they did not want her to "lose hope."

Ms. A described a close relationship with her parents when she was growing up and felt a great need to support them through their financial and other difficulties. She was an altruistic and other-directed person in both her personal and professional life and derived great satisfaction from being able to support others. Her professional work focused on the problems of new immigrants and on locating appropriate housing for them. She felt fulfilled by this work but feared that she might soon become unable to continue with it. Ms. A's husband suffered from a chronic medical condition, and her greatest concern was how he would manage without her. Her scores on the psychometric measures indicated a low level of depression but significant distress about dying and death, largely related to her concern about the burden on others. Her scores on the Experiences in Close Relationships Scale indicated a high level of attachment avoidance.

The Initial Session: Living With Waiting and Uncertainty

Ms. A presented in the first session as an articulate, well-groomed woman who looked well and who clearly described the story of her disease and its treatment. She reported many positive events that had occurred in her family life in the last few years but also acknowledged that the last two years had been "pretty rough" due to the various treatments and side effects that she had experienced. Although she believed that she had derived some benefit from these treatments, she had been removed from the last clinical trial because her disease had recurred. For the first time in the preceding two years, she was not currently enrolled in a clinical trial. Consequently, she felt it even more difficult to be "living with waiting and uncertainty." However, despite a prolonged and difficult disease course, Ms. A was calm in her demeanor and demonstrated no evident distress. This contradiction was puzzling, but perhaps consistent with her tendency to minimize her distress and to focus on the needs of others.

Despite her difficulties with her disease, Ms. A continued to be a compliant patient and a supportive caregiver for her family. In the initial CALM session, she dutifully provided information about her life, her disease, and her treatment but did not seem to be asking for anything for herself. It was unclear after this first meeting whether Ms. A would develop a deeper connection to the therapist or to her own inner life. Her focus on others and her self-reliant minimization of distress raised the question of whether there was silent despair and what would happen if her condition passed the "tipping point."

The Middle Sessions: Being Known

Although the first session seemed more cognitive than emotional, Ms. A had been watchful of the therapist and subsequently reported that the attention and interest that she experienced was profoundly meaningful for her. Although she tended to accommodate the needs of others and be "a good patient," she found it distressing to feel invisible as a person in the cancer clinics. She noted, "People don't read the charts or know who I am as a person or as a professional." As a result, she reported feeling "reduced to my illness, my treatment, and my symptoms." Feeling known in the CALM sessions was experienced as a great relief, which she said was "particularly important when you are already struggling with the loss of identity." The therapist's quiet, empathic listening was a new and important experience for Ms. A. This receptive approach had a restorative effect on her and helped to strengthen the therapeutic relationship on which Ms. A would later come to rely.

The Later Sessions: "I Am Dying"

Ms. A presented much differently in the fourth CALM session. Her voice was broken as she said that she was glad to see the therapist because she had received news that there were new lesions in her liver and lung and that no further anticancer treatment was available. When asked what she took this to mean, Ms. A said, "that I'm dying." This was a dramatic moment in the session, when a simple enquiry about Ms. A's interpretation of the news she had received led her to talk about the deepest fears that she had harbored about her condition. She said she had felt from the beginning that "my body holds the seeds of my own destruction." Ms. A had been unable to communicate this belief to anyone. To some extent, she had pursued ongoing cancer treatment to maintain hope for her family and to be a good patient for her oncology team. Ms. A was frightened about the future, but in some respects felt relief in no longer having to manage her fears entirely on her own.

The shift in her disease course and the deepening of the therapeutic relationship allowed Ms. A to think about different ways that she could manage her disease. She had thought of chemotherapy and participation in clinical trials as a "quality improvement project" and had viewed not receiving further treatment as "giving in." As a form of mentalization, the therapist reframed "giving in" as a psychological state rather than a fact of not receiving chemotherapy and suggested that it was perhaps now time to "shift the project" to focus on herself rather than on the disease. This intervention had a liberating effect on Ms. A, who now felt able to think about the benefits that she might receive from seeing the specialists in palliative care.

Attachment security had developed in the treatment process, which allowed Ms. A to express her fears and to feel that she could rely on another, rather than always needing to be the protector and supporter of others. Ms. A participated in one more clinical trial, which was unsuccessful, but then decided not to accept a subsequent trial that was offered. Her family was supportive of this decision.

The Final Session: Finding a Home

In the last session, Ms. A shared that CALM meant to her what a home would mean for a homeless person. She appreciated that the sessions provided the "time and space" to discuss existential issues in a way that she had not experienced before. She said that feeling known as a person in the sessions was profoundly meaningful to her and was a great benefit of CALM. Finding attachment security and reclaiming her sense of identity allowed Ms. A to assume a greater sense of agency in her treatment decisions. She became better able to communicate her concerns to her family and to accept support from them. She was also able to reach out to her professional community and allow them to honor her.

Ms. A's disease progressed over the next few months, and her life ended peacefully in her home with her family at her bedside. It seems likely that, in some way, CALM helped to ensure that her life ended in a way that she had wanted.

CASE SUMMARY: HOUSECLEANING AND MORTALITY

Ms. C, a 75-year-old married woman with advanced lung cancer, was referred to CALM for help with "future coping." The disease had metastasized by the time it was diagnosed, and she reported feeling that her "future was indeterminate." Ms. C was an energetic, action-oriented person who was uncomfortable with passivity and distressing emotions, a characteristic that seemed to have emerged from childhood experiences in which there was little room for her to explore or express her emotions. She expressed worry about her husband becoming depressed. He was a quieter, more introspective person who felt sad and vulnerable as a child and who viewed his wife as his protector. While he worried that her disease had taken some of the joy of living from her, she worried that her disease was causing suffering for him. Although he valued authentic communication from his wife, she believed that hearing her fears would overwhelm him. On the psychometric measures, Ms. C's measurement scores indicated low levels of depression but high levels of death anxiety and attachment avoidance.

The Initial Session: The Urgency of Housecleaning

Ms. C and her husband were a close unit and attended all CALM sessions together. In the initial session, she reported that her condition had been relatively stable, although she had a cough that troubled her. She tended to direct her attention to her husband whom she worried would become depressed if her disease progressed. She also felt an urgency to clean her house and to have things in order. It became evident, even in this first session, that Ms. C's focus on organizing things in her house was implicitly related to her fears about mortality and helplessness in the face of disease progression, represented in the fourth CALM domain.

The Middle Sessions

Ms. C's sense of urgency about getting their house in order began to feel overwhelming to her. Although she believed that she was preparing the house so that her husband would not be overwhelmed by this task after she died, he did not share her concerns. The middle CALM sessions allowed for Ms. C's focus on housecleaning to be mentalized. She began to accept that her strong urge to organize their home was related, in part, to her need to take concrete action in response to the uncontrollable threat of her cancer. Disentangling the fear of dying from the more practical desire to get their house in order and recognizing that she and her husband had different ways of responding to the threat of mortality allowed them to work together on a plan of action. This renegotiation of their attachment relationship, an aspect of the second CALM domain, was further propelled by their mutual perception that time was short.

Over the course of the middle sessions, another meaning of Ms. C's focus on her belongings emerged. She viewed some of the objects that they had inherited and collected over the years as an important part of her legacy. She wanted herself and her deceased parents to be remembered respect-fully, which was represented in her wish to have their belongings passed down to others who might value them.

Ms. C came to accept that the urgency of her focus on housecleaning was partly related to her tendency to take action in response to threat and to displace her internal concerns onto the external world or onto others. It was also related to the importance of having a legacy by which she and her parents would be remembered. Mentalizing these multiple meanings allowed them to be addressed throughout therapy and for her and her husband to negotiate how they would deal with them.

Emerging Double Awareness

As the sessions progressed, Ms. C was increasingly able to explore issues related to mortality, which allowed for double awareness to emerge. She thought of all the songs that she would like to have played at her funeral, wanting there to be some with sadness and others with joy. She hoped that she would be missed and that there would be some tears at her funeral, but also that there would be singing and dancing. She wanted to be remembered as someone who honored life, even in the face of a dreadful diagnosis. This double awareness became more prominent in later CALM sessions and was increasingly evident in the way that Ms. C and her husband chose to continue living their lives.

The Final Session: The Non-Ending

When Ms. C and her husband first began CALM, they believed that her survival would be very short-lived. This belief added a sense of urgency to the sessions, which allowed productive change to occur in a relatively short period of time. Fortuitously, her disease had an unexpectedly positive response to immunotherapy and stabilized. The CALM sessions ended with the understanding that Ms. C and her husband would return if and when her cancer progressed. Meanwhile, the therapy allowed them to live in a calmer, more satisfying way that they had not initially expected would be possible.

CASE SUMMARY: THE CONSIDERATE YOUNG WOMAN

Ms. P was a 35-year-old single woman with metastatic cervical cancer who was randomized to receive CALM as part of our large randomized controlled trial. She had been living at home with her father and her younger brother and was working as a manager of a small houseware store. Her parents had an acrimonious divorce when she was quite young. Ms. P often found herself acting as the liaison between them and was torn by her loyalties to both. Her scores on the psychometric measures before initiation of CALM indicated a moderate level of depressive symptoms and distress about dying and death, largely related to loss of opportunities and her future. Her scores on the attachment measure demonstrated higher attachment avoidance than on attachment anxiety.

The Initial Session: "I'm Coping Okay—The Problem Is Everyone Else"

In the first CALM session, Ms. P became tearful, before any words were spoken. She acknowledged that she had a lot to say and that she had not yet had a chance to speak to anyone about what she was feeling. She had just been informed in an earlier meeting with the oncologist that there had been progression of her bone metastases. Her oncologist seemed puzzled that this news was so upsetting to her because her disease had metastasized to bone at diagnosis. However, it was not until this clinic appointment that she fully realized that her cancer was incurable. She felt unsupported by her father whom she felt was pushing her to tell him about the news that she had received when she only wanted to be left alone in her sadness and grief.

Over the course of the session, Ms. P calmed and, with minimal prompting, described the challenges of her current treatment, her fears for her parents and their inability to cope with her disease and possible death, and her wish for a romantic partner with whom to face her cancer. She expressed deep regret that she had postponed trying to find a partner after she was diagnosed, assuming she would have time in the future to find someone to marry and with whom to have a family.

Ms. P tended to focus on the emotional needs of her parents and of others, who were sad that someone so young should be facing such a serious cancer. This attention to the emotional state of others was accompanied by difficulties in knowing what she thought and felt. The empathic but nonintrusive interest that the therapist demonstrated in the first session was the beginning of Ms. P's experience of the sessions as a "secure base," where she could understand herself without feeling overwhelmed and where she could plan for the time she had left. She agreed to bring a family caregiver—her brother—to the next CALM session.

The Middle Session: "I'll Run Interference For You"

Ms. P arrived to the session with her brother in good spirits, indicating that her radiation therapy was going well. They joked and talked easily together, describing the differing reactions of their family members to her cancer. Her brother was an outgoing person who said he had always enjoyed the attention of Ms. P, his older sister. This led to a discussion of Ms. P's tendency to focus on the needs of others and an acknowledgment that caring for her family had perhaps limited her independence and ability to establish her own romantic relationships. Both acknowledged that after their parents divorced, her father tended to rely on Ms. P as his companion and confidante. Without prompting, her brother offered to attend more to the feelings of their father and mother, reassuring Ms. P that they would be taken care of even if her illness progressed and she became unable to support them in the way she always had.

The Final Session: Wishes Understood and Expressed

Ms. P's cancer spread faster than was anticipated and within a few months of the first session, she was admitted to our inpatient palliative care unit for pain management. During that admission, a family session was arranged with both parents and all siblings in attendance. This was a highly emotional session in which everyone, at some point or another, became overwhelmed with emotion and unable to speak. Drawing on their comments about Ms. P and her role in the family, the therapist articulated how Ms. P experienced her role in the family. Her compassion and tendency "to think about everyone else's feelings first" was acknowledged by everyone in the family as a great strength, and Ms. P was able to say how much she now appreciated being the recipient of support. Her parents were able to set aside their differences and shortly after discharge, Ms. P died at her mother's home with her father in attendance.

BRIEFER CASE EXAMPLES

The case summaries described above highlight how CALM therapy may unfold over time. Next, briefer case examples illustrate specific challenges that frequently arise in the delivery of CALM.

Case Example: The Focus on a Single Domain

A 44-year-old man with metastatic melanoma began CALM with significant symptoms of depression and anxiety, which he attributed to the recent loss of a six-year relationship. In this and subsequent sessions, the patient seemed to focus solely on the relationship loss and to be unable or unwilling to reflect upon other domains. The therapist feared that the relationship issue, represented in the second CALM domain, was being explored at the expense of the three other domains. When she brought this case to group supervision, it became evident that issues related to all four CALM domains had been collapsed into this singular focus. The patient's preoccupation with the loss of his partner had been heightened by his awareness of the shortness of time. Moreover, his sense of meaning in life and his ability to make treatment decisions were limited by the lack of a life partner. The therapist allowed the patient to linger on the loss of the relationship, and cancer-related issues of CALM gradually emerged more explicitly over subsequent sessions.

This case example highlights the interrelationship of the CALM domains and the need for the therapist to allow patients to focus on the issues that are most important to them in the moment. The attunement and patience of the therapist allowed a more secure therapeutic attachment relationship to emerge, which then facilitated exploration of issues related to all four CALM domains.

Case Example: Self-Knowledge

A 50-year-old woman was in treatment for metastatic cervical cancer. She had been raised by a single mother who put great emphasis on the importance of physical appearance and who had always seemed to be emotionally needy. The patient wanted to "stay positive" in the face of her cancer and often laughed and smiled when describing hurtful scenarios with her mother. She avoided discussion of cancer or the possibility of dying and death. In response, the therapist often felt disengaged from the patient and bored and frustrated by their sessions.

The therapist sought to connect more deeply to the inner experience of the patient and to make use of her own experience. She commented on instances when the patient's emotional state was incongruous with the content of her conversation or when the patient showed hints of more authentic emotion. This approach allowed the patient to attend more closely to her emotional life and to explore feelings of disappointment and frustration related to her childhood experience. It became evident that the frustrations and disappointments related to her treatment course and disease progression had layered onto the feelings related to her early life experience. The CALM treatment process allowed the patient to explore these feelings and her fears about the adequacy of support as her disease progressed.

Case Example: Beneath the Surface

A 66-year-old man with metastatic prostate cancer was referred for CALM at the urging of his wife. In the initial CALM session, the patient reported that he had not asked his oncology team about his prognosis, that he preferred not to think about it, and that he had no distress or worry about what lay ahead. However, his scores on the Death and Dying Distress Scale indicated high levels of distress about future suffering and burden on his loved ones. Subsequent review of these scores with the patient led to a discussion of these fears, which could then be normalized and validated, and to an exploration of what had made it challenging for him to discuss them in therapy. He indicated that he had found thinking about the future to be overwhelming but that he hoped that reporting them on the measure would encourage the therapist to find a way to address them.

This case emphasizes the clinical value of collecting psychometric measure scores, which may allow for sensitive issues that patients may be initially reluctant to raise to emerge in the therapy.

Case Example: Facing the End

A 50-year-old man with metastatic sarcoma was experiencing difficulty with treatment decisions and was struggling to balance the needs of his second wife with those of his adult children from his first marriage. He engaged in CALM for the agreed upon six sessions and was able to explore and address issues in all four domains. In the sixth session, the patient reported that he felt supported, understood, and better able to manage his stressors. However, when the therapist summarized the gains the patient had made in therapy and the stability of his present situation, the patient responded by saying, "I feel like you're telling me that the therapy is finished now. I have found our sessions so helpful to me. I don't want them to end." The therapist felt distressed and conflicted about the termination, although the patient was in no other immediate distress.

When the training therapist brought this termination difficulty to the supervision group, it became evident that the termination of CALM had activated attachment anxiety in the patient, who feared what might lie ahead. This triggered feelings of guilt in the therapist about abandoning the patient at a time when he might still need support. The group encouraged the therapist to acknowledge the distress they were both feeling in the face of the limitations of time. The possibility of future "booster sessions" was also emphasized so that the patient and therapist did not need to say goodbye, understanding instead that further support could be available if necessary. This allowed the patient to accept the end of therapy and feel confident that further help would be available when it was needed.

Case Example: Recognizing the Tipping Point

A 44-year-old woman with metastatic breast cancer was referred for CALM when she developed bony pelvic metastases. She was tearful and distressed in the first CALM session about this complication and talked at length about her fears associated with the possibility of dying. What was most distressing to her was the thought of leaving behind her six-year-old daughter and husband. Subsequent radiation treatment to her hip relieved her pain and disability, and she began to contemplate returning to work as a teacher. The relief of her physical symptoms had led to a reduction of her distress and a wish to focus on living and not to think about her disease. The patient and the therapist agreed to suspend further CALM sessions until her clinical condition changed.

This case highlights that some patients with advanced disease who tend to be avoidant may not wish to begin or continue therapy unless their symptoms and disease course create distress that seems unmanageable. The flexibility of the CALM framework and the open-door approach of the therapist allow patients to postpone or suspend CALM and to resume when the need arises.

Case Example: Single Awareness

A 39-year-old woman recently diagnosed with metastatic lung cancer presented for CALM with significant anxiety and multiple concerns about her disease and treatment. These included fears about the side effects of planned chemotherapy, the impact of the disease on her children, and the long-standing tension in her relationship with her husband. She believed that her cancer was caused by her tendency to be pessimistic and negative. She linked her tendency to assume personal responsibility to her cultural background, which she said did not encourage counseling or emotional expression as a legitimate means to resolving personal difficulties. In the initial session, she explained that her goals were to gain control of her anger and negative thinking, and she hoped that the therapist would provide techniques to help her avoid negative thoughts.

The therapist explored the patient's belief that she was to blame for her cancer, but the patient held firmly to the idea that positive thinking might cure her disease. In response to the therapist's attempts to mentalize her situation and to suggest these ideas were feelings and not facts, the patient looked uncomfortable and became quiet. Prior to the second CALM session, this patient called to cancel explaining she had found a program at another hospital that was more in line with her therapeutic goals.

This case highlights the unsuitability of CALM for patients who are reluctant to reflect and wish only to think positively about their situation. For such individuals, a reflective therapy is either entirely unwanted or unsuitable, and double awareness is not a goal that they wish to pursue.

CONCLUSION

Although each CALM case is unique, the summaries and examples presented in this chapter indicate some of the common issues and challenges that may arise in CALM therapy. They also illustrate the potential clinical value of the psychometric measures and of group supervision.

Epilogue

The momentum of CALM has been importantly sustained by our international colleagues and collaborators. The first international collaboration was initiated with Anja Mehnert-Theuerkauf, PhD, Professor and Chair of the Department of Medical Psychology and Medical Sociology, University Medical Center, University of Leipzig, Leipzig, and her team in Germany, who have since conducted a large randomized controlled trial of CALM. This collaboration was followed by the introduction of CALM to Italy by Luigi Grassi, MD, Professor and Chair of Psychiatry, University of Ferrara, Department of Neurosciences and Rehabilitation, and Director, Hospital University Psychiatry Unit, S. Anna Hospital/ Local Health Trust, Ferrara, and Rosangela Caruso, MD, PhD, Associate Professor of Psychiatry, Institute of Psychiatry, University of Ferrara. Since then, collaborations have developed with China, led by Lili Tang, MD, Professor and Director, Department of Psycho-Oncology, Beijing Cancer Hospital, Beijing Institute for Cancer Research; President, Chinese Psycho-Oncology Society (CPOS), and Ying Pang, PhD, Clinical Psychologist, Department of Psycho-Oncology Beijing Cancer Hospital, Beijing; the Netherlands, led by Froukje de Vries, MD, PhD, Psychiatrist, the Netherlands Cancer Institute, Amsterdam, and An Reyners, MD, Professor of Palliative Medicine, Medical Oncologist, Department of Medical Oncology, University of Groningen, University Medical Center Groningen; Taiwan, led by Yeong-Yuh Juang, MD, Deputy Chief, Department of Palliative Medicine; Attending Psychiatrist, Department of Psychiatry, Koo Foundation Sun Yat-Sen Cancer Center; and President, Taiwan Psycho-Oncology Society; South Korea, led by Jungmin Woo, MD, PhD, Associate Professor, Department of Psychiatry, Kyungpook National

University School of Medicine, Daegu; Hong Kong, led by Wendy Lam, RN, PhD, FFPH, Associate Professor, School of Public Health; Director, Jockey Club Institute of Cancer Care, Li Ka Shing Faculty of Medicine, The University of Hong Kong; Portugal, led by Luzia Travado, PhD, Clinical Health Psychologist and Head of Psycho-Oncology, Clinical Center of the Champalimaud Centre for the Unknown, Champalimaud Foundation, Lisbon; the state of Virginia in the United States of America, led by Ashlee Loughan, PhD, Clinical Neuropsychologist; Assistant Professor of Neurology, School of Medicine, Virginia Commonwealth University and Massey Cancer Center, Virginia; Israel, led by David Hausner, MD, Head, Palliative Care Service, Sheba Medical Center, Ramat Gan, and Iris Gluck, MD, Head of Supportive and Palliative Care, Cancer Center at Sheba-Tel HaShomer Hospital Ramat Gan; Chile, led by Loreto Fernández González, MPH, Dalla Lana School of Public Health, University of Toronto (PhD candidate), Toronto, Canada, and Instituto Oncologico Fundación Arturo López Perez, Santiago; the Canadian province of Alberta, led by Janet de Groot, MD, Staff Psychiatrist, Tom Baker Cancer Centre; Professor, Cumming School of Medicine, University of Calgary, Calgary, Alberta; Jordan, led by Omar Shamieh, MD, Chairman, Department of Palliative Care, King Hussein Cancer Centre, Amman, and Ghadeer Al-Arjeh, MD, Senior Palliative Researcher and Instructor, Center for Palliative and Cancer Care in Conflict (CPCCC), King Hussein Cancer Center, Amman; Australia, led by Maria Ftanou, PhD, Lead Clinical Psychologist, Peter MacCallum Cancer Centre, Melbourne; Mexico, led by Alejandra Platas, Master in Neuropsychology, Clinical Psychologist, Department of Research and Breast Tumors, Instituto Nacional de Cancerología, Mexico City; and Joven y Fuerte: Program for the Care and Research of Young Women with Breast Cancer in Mexico, Mexico City; Japan, led by Ken Shimizu, MD, Chief, Department of Psycho-Oncology, Cancer Institute Hospital, Tokyo; and United Kingdom, initially involving Anne Lanceley, PhD, Senior Lecturer in Women's Cancer, Department of Women's Cancer, Institute for Women's Health, and Honorary Clinical Nurse Specialist, University College London Hospitals (UCLH), Gynaecological Cancer Centre, London, Sue Gessler, PhD, Consultant Clinical Psychologist, UCLH, Gynaecological Cancer Centre, and Honorary Senior Lecturer, Department of Women's Cancer, Institute for Women's Health, and Christian Schulz-Quach, MD, Assistant Professor, Department of Psychiatry, University of Toronto, and Staff Psychiatrist, University Health Network, Centre for Mental Health, Toronto, Canada. To give voice to their experiences of CALM, some of their comments are included below.

The first time I heard about CALM therapy was when attending a lecture given by Dr. Gary Rodin at the 2017 IPOS [International Psycho-Oncology Society] World Congress in Berlin. I was impressed by CALM's comprehensive structure and holistic psychosocial approach covering all domains of human suffering for patients with advanced or metastatic cancer. However, I questioned whether CALM, yet another psychosocial intervention developed by Western therapists, could fit into Eastern culture. I decided I had to attend the CALM workshop the following year. After completing the workshop, I had no doubts. Gary and Sarah demonstrated how CALM therapy can have an impact by simply creating a space for patients to express their concerns and distress while covering issues such as physical symptoms, close relationships, meaning, hope, and mortality. As a mental health professional working at a cancer center, I have wanted and have tried to intervene when patients feel distress. In traditional Taiwanese culture, people understand the idea of yin and yang, living and dying—this is how the universe works. However, it is still difficult to openly discuss with patients the balance of death and dying and living in the present moment. CALM therapy creates the openness and opportunity to talk about these issues. Just as Laozi said in the Tao Te Ching, "The Tao never strives, yet nothing is left undone." That is what CALM therapy is.

—Yeong-Yuh Juang, CALM Site Lead (Taiwan)

Working with advanced cancer patients used to be a dreaded challenge for me before I learned of CALM. I was never sure what patients and I should discuss during the consultations. In Chinese culture, family members usually withhold bad news from the patients in order to preserve their sense of hope. As a result, so many patients were unclear about their diagnosis or prognosis, and their family members often wanted me, the psychotherapist, to encourage patients to stay optimistic and to insist on continuing to receive treatment.

When I struggled to find a solution, CALM let me see the light. I began to conduct my consultations with patients with advanced cancer following the framework outlined in CALM. I was surprised to find it was effective with my patients, even though it was developed in the West. Even patients who are unclear about their diagnosis or prognosis are tortured by their disease. They feel as though their lives are shortened, worry that they have no future, and are afraid of being a burden to their family. Exploring with patients the four domains of CALM allowed me to connect with these individuals and helped my patients reconnect with their real lives and their families. Death and dying does not feel like a taboo topic anymore. I find some patients are willing to talk about death, as long as I am prepared to offer them an opportunity to talk about it.

—Ying Pang, CALM Site (Beijing)

My first encounter with CALM was in the fall of 2017, when Dr. Gary Rodin visited our cancer center in the Netherlands. Beyond resonating well with our clinical practice, CALM provided a theoretical framework with scientific evidence to support its effectiveness. As a result, we decided to board the international CALM train. Since then, our efforts to use CALM in Dutch cancer care have focused on integrated clinical implementation and research. This has helped us as clinicians to better understand CALM therapy and will provide evidence and guidance to support further implementation.

One important lesson we have learned is that a team of motivated therapists is not enough to start a CALM program. Leadership, dedicated time, and funding were key ingredients for successful implementation at our site. Leadership was essential to prioritize and to advocate for the project within the hospital. A clinical and research coordinator was necessary to motivate and facilitate clinicians carrying a high workload already. And finally, funding helped to pay for dedicated time and to compensate for the startup costs of the project.

The collaboration with the CALM developers and the international CALM community helped to spearhead the project. The international collaborations and workshops have been some of the most inspirational parts of the journey so far. It is particularly striking that when therapists from very different cultures share their patients' stories, they are so remarkably similar. The universal applicability of CALM and its global uptake indicate a high need for CALM and are, to me, as convincing as the efficacy shown with the trial data.
　　　　—Froukje de Vries, CALM Site Lead (the Netherlands)

CALM outlines several important therapeutic ingredients. However, one that has struck me as particularly impressive and beautiful while implementing CALM in South Korea is the notion of "co-thinking." Under the atmosphere of the therapist and patient working together, important changes can occur. In this secure attachment relationship with the therapist, patients feel less anxious and can think more widely and deeply. Patients may begin to see death from various perspectives and realize that there might be life in death and death in life. They can start to broaden their fixed and painful ideas of death. Consequently, they can begin living meaningfully again.

During CALM, one of my patients told me, "This was my first experience with advanced cancer since I was born, literally. Really, it was a very new situation to me. So, it was natural that I did not have an answer for this. And it was natural that you did not know everything. But we have tried to find the answer together . . . The answer has changed from time to time, but my memories and feelings of being together are helping me feel comfortable . . . And now I can explore another way of thinking and know that considering different perspectives can help to make me comfortable."

Though it is not ever easy to find the right answers in these heavy situations, CALM has provided me with a very precious clue.
　　　　—Jungmin Woo, CALM Site Lead (South Korea)

As a neuropsychologist and quality of life expert working alongside patients with neurological cancers, I am extremely aware of the heightened distress experienced by those with advanced cancer. In fact, for years I struggled with the paucity of evidenced-based treatment regimens available for terminally ill populations. CALM has finally provided a framework specifically targeting our patients' needs.

I began my training in CALM approximately two years ago. I recall attending my first workshop and feeling relief that a global team was bringing to light the concerns my patients were facing. And now, we have an established evidenced-based practice for not only relief, but the prevention of their symptoms. Since implementing CALM in my neuro-oncology clinic, I have witnessed many brain tumor patients confront their greatest fears (i.e., disease progression & mortality) with increased acceptance and dignity. I have heard patients say: "It is nice to speak with someone who is comfortable with the topic of death," "Though difficult discussions, you have helped me prepare for the end of my life," and "This program has supported me in my greatest time of need." As I prepare to formally adapt CALM for brain cancer patients, my hope is that CALM will become standard of care for all advanced cancer patients internationally. The challenges faced by those with terminal illness are universal and CALM has targeted both the principle concepts and processes aimed to assist patients in finding meaning while navigating their inevitable mortality.

Our patients are distressed. Our patients need help. We finally have a resource available in CALM.

—Ashlee Loughan, CALM Site Lead (Virginia, USA)

A diagnosis of advanced cancer can be very frightening for patients and their families. Patients and their spouses have been found to experience high rates of depression, anxiety, hopelessness, demoralization, uncertainty, and a loss of self and identity. Many patients with advanced disease do not receive psychological interventions. Managing Cancer and Living Meaningfully (CALM) is a short-term therapeutic intervention that can help to reduce distress and symptom burden and optimize quality of life. CALM provides patients and family members with an opportunity to address treatment concerns, improve communication with their treating team, adjust and renegotiate changes in their personal relationships, reflect on what is meaningful, and face their fears associated with death and dying.

Our Melbourne, Australia "CALM team" includes psychologists, social workers, psychiatrists, mental health nurses, and a clinical nurse specialist. Our team attended introductory and advanced training and has met with other global CALM clinicians. We receive monthly supervision from Gary Rodin and are committed to the continued development of our clinical CALM skills. The supervision is always supportive. It offers us a safe place to better understand the underlying theory and CALM techniques, to refine

CALM to suit our population and clinical setting, and to reflect on any process issues or challenges experienced by clinicians who work with people at the end of life.

CALM is an evidenced-based intervention that can assist patients to live well and with hope while facing the challenges associated with dying.
—Maria Ftanou, CALM Site Lead (Australia)

The Italian experience with CALM started in 2012, when we took part in a CALM workshop at the Princess Margaret Cancer Centre in Toronto. Since that time, our team, which is part of a wider project coordinated by the Institute of Psychiatry at the University of Ferrara focused on psychotherapy in oncology and palliative care and on person-centered medicine, has continued to attend CALM workshops, to develop our interest in CALM, and to contribute to the CALM initiative.

With the intention of exploring the feasibility of CALM in the Italian cultural context, we recently carried out the first pilot CALM study in Italy (Caruso, Sabato, et al., 2020). Our findings were promising: qualitative analyses showed that CALM was positively accepted by Italian patients with advanced cancer, who indicated finding benefit in the construction of a shared reflective space in which the therapist facilitated discussions about death and dying, loss, spirituality, relationships with significant others, and concerns related to the aftermath of death. Furthermore, quantitative analyses suggested that CALM has the potential to reduce levels of depression, death anxiety, and general anxiety, and to increase levels of post-traumatic growth. These results encouraged us to design the first CALM randomized controlled trial in Italy, which is ongoing and involves the University Centres of Ferrara and Turin (Caruso, Nanni, et al., 2020).

In 2017, the first Italian CALM workshop was organized at the University of Ferrara with the assistance of Gary Rodin and Carmine Malfitano. The workshop, which aimed to introduce CALM to Italian physicians, psychotherapists, nurses, and other figures working in advanced cancer settings was very well received by clinicians from all over the country.

In the last years, the Italian experience of CALM was presented at several international scientific congresses (e.g., International Psycho-Oncology Society Congress, Lisbon 2014 and Berlin 2017; the European Association of Psychosomatic Medicine, Verona, 2018; the International College of Psychosomatic Medicine, Florence, 2019). The University of Ferrara is now part of the Global Institute of Psychosocial, Palliative and End-of-Life Care (GIPPEC) and the network of collaborators of the Global CALM Program, which aims to develop scientific evidence with respect to CALM in diverse settings and to implement CALM as a standard of care for patients facing advanced cancer.
—Rosangela Caruso and Luigi Grassi, CALM Site Leads (Italy)

In our palliative and hospice care practice, we tend to see less open communication among patients and healthcare providers related to feelings, concerns, and fears. This is likely due to cultural factors as well as a lack of psychosocial and spiritual care training for healthcare disciplines. However, King Hussein Cancer Center (KHCC), home of the largest comprehensive palliative care program in Jordan, recognizes the importance of having multidimensional and holistic care for patients and families. As such, in 2018, the first CALM workshop was conducted at KHCC by Dr. Gary Rodin. The workshop included practical and theoretical aspects and was attended by an interdisciplinary team of doctors, nurses, psychologists, social workers, and clinical pharmacists. The workshop was eye opening and our team agreed that CALM could be a practical and valuable option for a large portion of our patients with advanced cancer. There was great enthusiasm among the palliative and psychosocial teams to pursue CALM therapy training, implementation, and research, as many studies supported the use of CALM therapy to relieve psychological and spiritual suffering for patients facing advanced disease.

To translate enthusiasm into action, a group of five health care professionals from KHCC attended an advanced CALM workshop in London in July 2019. The workshop covered CALM therapy principles and practice in depth and included live simulation training. This was a life-changing experience and encouraged the team to further advance CALM therapy at KHCC. Following this training in London, the team started to recruit patients and apply CALM therapy under the supervision of Gary Rodin and his CALM team. One of our CALM therapists reported, "I tried to cover all elements of CALM therapy to support my patient and I was surprised by the abundance of shared personal private information. I felt our patients are starving to find someone who can listen to them." Another said, "Patients are very grateful, and they have started to look at things from a different point of view." Patients reported that CALM therapy was helpful in many ways, including in relieving their anxiety and fears and in improving their relationships and their communication with family members and others. Our healthcare professionals felt that CALM gave them a sense of self-satisfaction for helping patients during this precious time. Though sometimes patients have difficulty keeping up with their therapy appointments due to sickness or transportation difficulties, we found that this therapy is both culturally and religiously acceptable.

Our plan moving forward includes training more staff in CALM, conducting collaborative research projects with GIPPEC to establish CALM's feasibility and effectiveness in Jordan, and establishing KHCC as a CALM regional center of excellence.
      —Omar Shamieh and Ghadeer Al-Arjeh, CALM Site Leads (Jordan)

The Jockey Club Institute of Cancer Care (LKS Faculty of Medicine, The University of Hong Kong) joined the Global CALM Program in 2018 and began the implementation of CALM therapy within our centre. We found that the flexibility of the CALM approach offered a platform for patients with advanced and metastatic cancer and their caregivers to discuss a diverse range of challenges with their health care professionals. Most importantly, these discussions need not be restricted to mental health specialists. This is especially beneficial in Hong Kong, as seeking mental health services remains strongly stigmatized in Eastern culture. Furthermore, the CALM intervention is suitable and feasible to be implemented in any stages throughout the illness trajectory, facilitating the early introduction of palliative care in advanced cancer care. Our next step is to evaluate the effectiveness of CALM in our local population, as well as introduce CALM into our medical training.

—Wendy Lam, CALM Site Lead (Hong Kong)

We have evaluated CALM in a pilot and a bi-center randomized controlled trial (RCT) at the University Medical Centers of Leipzig and Hamburg. Meanwhile we have implemented CALM in our routine outpatient and inpatient psycho-oncological care. Therapists' experiences with CALM have been very positive. The patients and caregivers rated CALM as supportive and helpful. The following factors contributed to improved psychological adjustment and disease management: a safe framework for disease processing, learning to cope with frightening feelings, learning to communicate better with relatives and the professional treatment team, and feeling empowered in making medical decisions. Our research indicates that CALM therapy is highly accepted by patients with advanced cancer, reduces psychological distress and improves patient's quality of life. Ongoing research activities include the implementation and evaluation of CALM as a web-based program.

— Anja Mehnert-Theuerkauf, CALM Site Lead (Germany)

We had been providing psychotherapy for advanced cancer patients in the Japanese oncology setting, but we did not have a standardized approach to this treatment. Becoming aware of this lack, we became interested in CALM and invited Dr. Gary Rodin to hold a CALM workshop in our cancer center in June, 2017. Through our experience in it, we came to believe that CALM would be useful in Japan, because it has a very flexible structure that fits with Japanese culture. We then decided to introduce CALM into our practice in Japan and started a valuable collaboration that has continued since that time. We are very thankful to Dr. Rodin and his colleagues for their extraordinary support. We have been happy to receive his supervision so often and some of us have learned the essence of CALM. We have now started a multicenter clinical trial to investigate the usefulness and feasibility of CALM in Japanese cancer patients. In the near future, many more Japanese psycho-oncologists will learn CALM and use it in clinical practice.

— Ken Shimizu, CALM Site Lead (Japan)

CALM is not just an evidence-based intervention. It is also a tool to engage in deep reflection on the nature of human suffering and hope with people who are traversing a difficult stage of their lives. As a clinician, CALM has not only provided a framework to work with when doing psychotherapy; it has also offered what is to date one of the most comprehensive approaches to understanding cancer and its uniqueness as an illness. In a field where medical jargon and the language of scientific evidence are dominant, having a clinical and theoretical framework that focuses on the individual and the human condition—without sacrificing technical rigor—has been key for my professional development.

My first encounter with CALM was in 2014 in Santiago, Chile, when I was as a recently graduated psychologist working in cancer care. Since then, CALM has shaped my practice and my own setting of values in terms of what I aim to do as a clinician and as an advocate for better access to palliative care. I have been extremely fortunate to continue my training in CALM and to develop amazing relationships with first class mentors and friends in Canada and globally. Gary, Sarah, and the staff at GIPPEC have set the standard of what psycho-oncology should look like, while building an inspiring community of clinicians from around the world of which I am happy and grateful to be a part of.

—Loreto Fernández González, CALM Site Lead (Chile)

The implementation process of CALM in our center has taken off gradually, beginning soon after attending the CALM workshop in Israel in 2019. Our experience so far has been incredibly positive. Several cases were referred to CALM therapy from our palliative care colleagues who attended the workshop. The first few cases were seen by our lead social worker alongside a palliative care nurse. This dual approach proved to be very useful for building the team's confidence in providing CALM therapy and provided an opportunity to relate to multiple aspects of the cancer experience – medical, psychosocial, and spiritual. The involvement of family members in some sessions has enriched the discussions and has helped them tremendously in coping with their loved one's illness.

Our team has received wonderful supervision from our CALM mentors at the Princess Margaret Cancer Centre, which has added significantly to our growing confidence in the method. We plan to continue the implementation process in Sheba and hope to involve more palliative care team members in providing CALM therapy.

We would like to deeply thank Gary Rodin, Sarah Hales, and all the team members who have been involved in developing CALM therapy. We are grateful for the wonderful opportunity to join CALM Global and implement the method in Israel.

—Iris Gluck MD, David Hausner MD, Dania Weber BA, and
Ruth Elkayam MA, CALM Site Leads (Israel)

In Alberta, Canada, we are implementing CALM through a research program that allows us to build on current linkages between psychosocial oncology and palliative care (Rodin,

An, et al., 2020). Peer supervision, with the opportunity to share experiences and theoretical perspectives as well as learn from global colleagues in virtual interprofessional communities of practice, is expected to deepen our clinical work.

We find that CALM's clear structure, with its four domains that help clinicians open up conversations about mortality and meaning with patients individually or together with their close other, makes CALM a valuable model for interested psychosocial, palliative care, and psychiatry clinicians and trainees.

We are particularly interested in the capacity of CALM to deepen communication in partner relationships when one has advanced cancer (Mah et al., 2020). Dr. Kathleen Sitter from the University of Calgary will bring the digital story-telling method ("Patient Stories," n.d.) to explore the close others' experience of CALM. The provision of story-telling through technology among women with breast cancer has enhanced healthcare practitioners' understanding of the patient experience of treatment. In the same way, as we implement CALM as part of our psychosocial oncology program, we hope to deepen our understanding of the close others' experience of CALM both individually and as part of a couple.

By writing this book, Dr. Rodin and Dr. Sarah Hales have performed an extremely valuable service for clinicians, therapists, and their patients.

—Janet de Groot, CALM Site Lead (Alberta, Canada)

REFERENCES

Caruso, R., Nanni, M. G., Rodin, G., Hales, S., Malfitano, C., De Padova, S., Bertelli, T., Belvederi Murri, M., Bovero, A., Miniotti, M., Leombruni, P., Zerbinati, L., Sabato, S., & Grassi, L. (2020). Effectiveness of a brief manualized intervention, Managing Cancer and Living Meaningfully (CALM), adapted to the Italian cancer care setting: Study protocol for a single-blinded randomized controlled trial. *Contemporary Clinical Trials Communications, 20*, 100661. doi: 10.1016/j.conctc.2020.100661.

Caruso, R., Sabato S., Nanni, M. G., Hales, S., Rodin, G., Malfitano, C., Tiberto, E., De Padova, S., Bertelli, T., Belvederi Murri, M., Zerbinati, L., & Grassi, L. (2020). Application of Managing Cancer and Living Meaningfully (CALM) in advanced cancer patients: An Italian pilot study. *Psychotherapy and Psychosomatics, 89*(6), 402–404.

Mah, K., Shapiro, G. K., Hales, S., Rydall, A., Malfitano, C., An, E., Nissim, R., Li, M., Zimmermann, C., & Rodin, G. (2020). The impact of attachment security on death preparation in advanced cancer: The role of couple communication. *Psycho-Oncology, 29*(5), 833–840.

Patient stories. (2020). https://www.patientstories.ca/

Rodin, G., An, E., Schnall, J., & Malfitano, C. (2020). Psychological interventions for advanced disease: Implications for oncology and palliative care. *Journal of Clinical Oncology, 38*(9), 885–904.

Death and Dying Distress Scale (DADDS)

Having cancer can bring to mind thoughts and feelings about life and death. Listed below are several thoughts or concerns that some people with cancer may think about, at any stage of their disease.

Please tell us how distressed you felt over the past 2 weeks about each item listed below. By distress, we refer generally to negative feelings such as being angry, afraid, sad, or anxious.

If you have many different negative feelings about an item, choose your answer based on the strongest negative feeling that you've had. Please circle only one number per line.

0 = I was not distressed about this thought or concern.
1 = I experienced very little distress.
2 = I experienced mild distress.
3 = I experienced moderate distress.
4 = I experienced great distress.
5 = I experienced extreme distress.

Over the past 2 weeks, how distressed did you feel about:

1. Not having done all the things that I wanted to do. 0 1 2 3 4 5
2. Not having said all that I wanted to say to the people 0 1 2 3 4 5
   I care about.

3. Not having achieved my life goals and ambitions. 0 1 2 3 4 5
4. Not knowing what happens near the end of life. 0 1 2 3 4 5
5. Not having a future. 0 1 2 3 4 5
6. The missed opportunities in my life. 0 1 2 3 4 5
7. Running out of time. 0 1 2 3 4 5
8. Being a burden to others. 0 1 2 3 4 5
9. The impact of my death on my loved ones. 0 1 2 3 4 5
10. My own death and dying. 0 1 2 3 4 5

Over the past 2 weeks, how distressed did you feel that your own death and dying may:

11. Happen suddenly or unexpectedly 0 1 2 3 4 5
12. Be prolonged or drawn out. 0 1 2 3 4 5
13. Happen when I am alone. 0 1 2 3 4 5
14. Happen with a lot of pain or suffering. 0 1 2 3 4 5
15. Happen very soon. 0 1 2 3 4 5

Re-printed with permission from *Lo, C., Hales, S., Zimmermann, C., Gagliese, L., Rydall, A., & Rodin, G. (2011). Measuring death-related anxiety in advanced cancer: Preliminary psychometrics of the Death and Dying Distress Scale. *Journal of Pediatric Hematology/Oncology, 33*(Suppl2), S140–S145. doi:10.1097/MPH.0b013e318230e1fd.
*Please see the Lo et al., 2011 article for scoring instructions.

Experiences in Close Relationships Scale–Modified Short Form (ECR-M16)

The following statements concern how you feel in close relationships with others. In the following statements the term 'other people' refers to people with whom you feel close. Using the rating scale, indicate how much you agree or disagree with each statement by circling *one (1) number per line*.

1	2	3	4	5	6	7
Disagree	...	...	Neutral	...	...	Agree

1. I get uncomfortable when other people want to be very close to me.

    1   2   3   4   5   6   7

2. I worry about being abandoned.

    1   2   3   4   5   6   7

3. I tell people with whom I feel close just about everything.

    1   2   3   4   5   6   7

4. I need a lot of reassurance that I am loved by people with whom I feel close.

    1   2   3   4   5   6   7

5. I don't feel comfortable opening up to other people.

    1   2   3   4   5   6   7

6. I worry a lot about my relationships.

          1   2   3   4   5   6   7

7. I usually discuss my problems and concerns with people with whom I feel close.

          1   2   3   4   5   6   7

8. I find that other people don't want to get as close as I would like.

          1   2   3   4   5   6   7

9. I try to avoid getting too close to other people

          1   2   3   4   5   6   7

10. I worry that other people won't care about me as much as I care about them.

          1   2   3   4   5   6   7

11. I don't mind asking other people for comfort, advice, or help.

          1   2   3   4   5   6   7

12. I get frustrated when other people are not around as much as I would like.

          1   2   3   4   5   6   7

13. I prefer not to be too close to other people.

          1   2   3   4   5   6   7

14. I worry a fair amount about losing people with whom I feel close.

          1   2   3   4   5   6   7

15. It helps to turn to other people in times of need.

          1   2   3   4   5   6   7

16. I resent it when people with whom I feel close spend time away from me.

          1   2   3   4   5   6   7

Reprinted with permission from *Lo, C., Walsh, A., Mikulincer, M., Gagliese, L., Zimmermann, C., & Rodin, G. (2009). Measuring attachment security in patients with advanced cancer: Psychometric properties of a modified and brief Experiences in Close Relationships scale. *Psycho-Oncology, 18*(5), 490–499. https://doi.org/10.1002/pon.1417
*Please see the Lo et al., 2009 article for scoring instructions.

Quality of Life at the End of Life–Cancer Scale (QUAL-EC)

I'd like you to think back over the last month. Please tell me the three physical or emotional symptoms that have bothered you the most during that time. Some examples are pain, nausea, lack of energy, confusion, depression, anxiety and shortness of breath.

Symptom #1: _____

Symptom #2: _____

Symptom #3: _____

If you have had no physical or emotional symptoms that bothered you over the last month, then skip to question #4.

Of the symptoms listed above, which one symptom has bothered you the most this past week?

_____

Please answer the following 3 questions based on this one symptom:

	Rarely	A few times	Fairly often	Very often	Most of the time
1. During the last week, how often have you experienced this symptom?	1	2	3	4	5

2. During the last week, on average, how severe has this symptom been?	Very mild	Mild	Moderate	Severe	Very severe
	1	2	3	4	5

3. During the last week, how much has this symptom interfered with your ability to enjoy life?	Not at all	A little bit	A moderate amount	Quite a bit	Completely
	1	2	3	4	5

Below is a list of statements that other people with an illness have said may be important. Please tell me how true each statement is for you.

1 = Not at all
2 = A little bit
3 = A moderate amount
4 = Quite a bit
5 = Completely

4. Although I cannot control certain aspects of my illness, I have a sense of control about my treatment decisions   1   2   3   4   5

5. I participate as much as I want in the decisions about my care   1   2   3   4   5

6. Beyond my illness, my doctor has a sense of who I am as a person   1   2   3   4   5

7. In general, I know what to expect about the course of my illness   1   2   3   4   5

8. As my illness progresses, I know where to go to get answers to my questions   1   2   3   4   5

9. I worry that my family is not prepared to cope with the future   1   2   3   4   5

10. At times, I worry that I will be a burden to my family   1   2   3   4   5

11. Thoughts of dying frighten me   1   2   3   4   5

12. I worry about the financial strain caused by my illness   1   2   3   4   5

13. I have been able to say important things to those close to me   1   2   3   4   5

14. I make a positive difference in the lives of others	1	2	3	4	5
15. I have been able to share important things with my family	1	2	3	4	5
16. Despite my illness, I have a sense of meaning in my life	1	2	3	4	5
17. There is someone in my life with whom I can share my deepest thoughts	1	2	3	4	5

Patient Health Questionnaire–9 (PHQ-9)

Over the _last 2 weeks_, how often have you been bothered by any of the following problems?

> 0 = Not at all
> 1 = Several days
> 2 = More than half the days
> 3 = Nearly every day

1. Little interest or pleasure in doing things	0	1	2	3
2. Feeling down, depressed, or hopeless	0	1	2	3
3. Trouble falling or staying asleep, or sleeping too much	0	1	2	3
4. Feeling tired or having little energy	0	1	2	3
5. Poor appetite or overeating	0	1	2	3
6. Feeling bad about yourself, or that you are a failure, or have let yourself or your family down	0	1	2	3
7. Trouble concentrating on things, such as reading the newspaper or watching television	0	1	2	3

8. Moving or speaking so slowly that other people could have noticed. Or the opposite–being so fidgety or restless that you have been moving around a lot more than usual   0   1   2   3

9. Thoughts that you would be better off dead, or of hurting yourself in some way   0   1   2   3

Total
Score   _____

9a**. Is there a chance you would do something to end your life?

Yes   ☐

No   ☐

10. If you checked off <u>any</u> problems, how <u>difficult</u> have these problems made it for you to do your work, take care of things at home, or get along with other people?

Not difficult at all   ☐
Somewhat difficult   ☐
Very difficult   ☐
Extremely difficult   ☐

CALM Treatment Integrity Measure (CTIM)

Therapist ID: _____

Patient ID: _____

Case Supervision Date (DD.MM.YYYY): _____

Completion Date (DD.MM.YYYY): _____

This evaluation is completed on the basis of the case discussion in group supervision and the therapist's skills as demonstrated in those sessions. Each case presented will have one evaluation form completed. If a skill was not employed in situations which demanded it, then the skill should be rated negatively. If a skill was not employed because it was not applicable, the item can be left blank.

1: Need improvement   2: Satisfactory   3: Excellent

The therapeutic relationship
____ Shows empathic understanding of patient experiences
____ Responds genuinely/honestly to patient thoughts and feelings
____ Promotes reflexive awareness (ability to consider multiple psychological responses to an event)
____ Acknowledges the realities of the patient's condition/situation
____ Maintains professional boundaries while engaging with patient experiences
____ Demonstrates investment/motivation/engagement in the therapeutic process

Modulating affect
___ Is able to appropriately modulate the emotional state of the patient
___ Demonstrates comfort with emotional distress
___ Helps increase patient ability to think about/manage negative emotions/events

Shifting frame
___ Shift between supportive, exploratory, and problem-solving therapeutic frames as necessary
___ Adjusts the content and timing of sessions based on the patient's physical and psychological state

Interpretations
___ Offers potential explanations for the patient's pattern of distress, thoughts, or behaviors
___ Offers interpretations in the spirit of dialogue and exchange between therapist and patient

Termination
___ Treatment ended with understanding of open-door policy; that therapist has not "given up" on patient

Rate the therapist's skills when addressing each domain, if applicable.

1: Need improvement   2: Satisfactory   3: Excellent

Symptom management and communication with healthcare providers
___ Encourages better understanding of disease
___ Encourages patient's active involvement in medical care
___ Promotes patient consideration of treatment options
___ Supports communication with healthcare providers

Changes in self and relations with close others
___ Explores patient feelings about their life history
___ Validates patient's sense of worth in light of their accomplishments
___ Acknowledges disappointments or regrets that the patient has experienced
___ Explores the relational changes imposed by disease
___ Explores fears and anxieties about dependency and loss of autonomy
___ Encourages appropriate communication and support-giving/taking from close others

Spirituality or sense of meaning and purpose

___ Explores the patient's spiritual beliefs and/or sense of meaning and purpose in life

___ Supports understanding of the personal meaning of their experience of suffering and dying

___ Evaluates priorities and goals in the face of advanced disease

___ Helps to create new meanings regarding the patient's life trajectory, goals, and suffering

Thinking of the future, hope, and mortality

___ Explores patient attitudes towards the future (i.e., hopes and fears about living and dying)

___ Allows expression of sadness and anxiety about the progression of disease

___ Explores feelings about death and dying

___ Promotes discussion of advance care planning

___ Helps to sustain realistic hope and engagement in life while acknowledging mortality

Reprinted with permission. © 2018. American Society of Clinical Oncology. All rights reserved. Rodin, G., Lo, C., Rydall, A., Shnall, J., Malfitano, C., Chiu, A., Panday, T., Watt, S., An, E., Nissim, R., Li, M., Zimmermann, C., & Hales, S. (2018). Managing Cancer and Living Meaningfully (CALM): A randomized controlled trial of a psychological intervention for patients with advanced cancer. *Journal of Clinical Oncology*, 36(23), 2422–2432. https://doi.10.1200/JCO.2017.77.1097.
*Since publication, the CTIM has been modified to include an additional competency: "Termination."

Clinical Evaluation Questionnaire (CEQ)–CALM

Please take a moment to think about your CALM therapy sessions. If an item below does not apply to you, please circle "**N/A**." Please circle only one number per line.

0 = Not at all
1 = A little bit
2 = Somewhat
3 = Quite a bit
4 = Very much

To what extent has your CALM therapy helped you to:

1. Freely discuss my concerns about cancer and my treatment options   N/A   0   1   2   3   4
2. Talk and feel understood how cancer has affected my life   N/A   0   1   2   3   4
3. Deal with changes in my relationships as a result of cancer   N/A   0   1   2   3   4
4. Explore better ways to communicate with my healthcare team, my family, and others   N/A   0   1   2   3   4
5. Clarify my values and beliefs   N/A   0   1   2   3   4
6. Talk about my concerns about the future and to be less frightened   N/A   0   1   2   3   4
7. Better express and manage my feelings   N/A   0   1   2   3   4

Please feel free to share any comments (positive or negative) about your CALM therapy:

_____

_____

_____

_____

_____

_____

_____

_____

_____

CALM Session 1 Therapy Notes

Therapist: _____

Patient ID: _____

Session Number: _____

Date: _____

Patient Identification (age, gender, cultural background, living arrangements, family/social constellation, employment, and financial supports)

_____

_____

_____

Cancer History (story of onset, diagnosis, treatment, course)

_____

_____

_____

Current Status (level of distress, current stressors, source of supports, methods of coping)

_____

_____

_____

Psychiatric History (diagnoses, treatment, history of suicidality/
homicidality)

_____
_____
_____

Developmental History (story of early family life, childhood, identity, relational functioning)

_____
_____
_____

Domain 1 – Symptom Management and Communication with Healthcare
Providers

_____
_____
_____

Domain 2 – Changes in Self and Relations with Close Others

_____
_____
_____

Domain 3 – Spirituality and the Sense of Meaning and Purpose

_____
_____
_____

Domain 4 – Preparing for the Future, Hope, and Mortality

_____
_____
_____

Therapeutic Process (relationship, affect regulation, reflective
functioning)

_____
_____
_____

Impression and Plan

_____

_____

_____

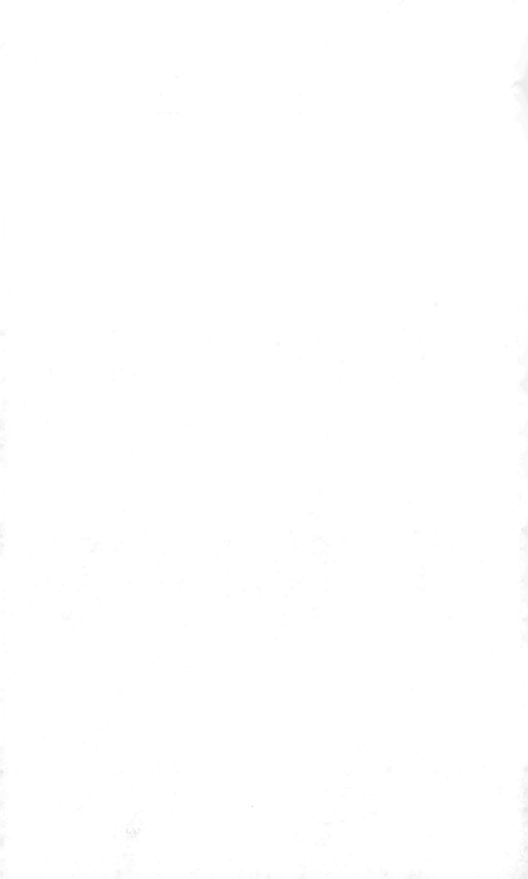

CALM Sessions 2–8 Therapy Notes

Therapist: _____

Patient ID: _____

Session Number: _____

Date: _____

Length: _____

Current Status (distress, stressors, supports, coping)

_____
_____
_____

Domain 1 – Symptom Management and Communication with Healthcare Providers

_____
_____
_____

Domain 2 – Changes in Self and Relations with Close Others

_____
_____
_____

Domain 3 – Spirituality and the Sense of Meaning and Purpose

_____

_____

_____

Domain 4 – Preparing for the Future, Hope, and Mortality

_____

_____

_____

Therapeutic Process (relationship, affect regulation, reflective functioning)

_____

_____

_____

Impression and Plan

_____

_____

_____

INDEX

Tables and figures are indicated by *t* and *f* following the page number.

balance of living and dying, 173
bargaining, in Kübler-Ross five-stage
    model, 32
barriers to optimal delivery of
    psychological care, 103–104
bereavement, 33
booster sessions, 194
borderline personality disorder, 54
Bowlby, J., 46, 47
Breitbart, W., 101
brooding, 93

Calhoun, L., 91
CALM. *See* Managing Cancer and Living
    Meaningfully
CALM supervisors, 125, 132
CALM therapists
    active ingredients of CALM process,
      150–154
    certification, 125, 132
    general discussion, 146–147
CALM Treatment Integrity Measure
    (CTIM), 115, 179, 217–219
CALM treatment manual. *See* treatment
    manual, CALM
cancer. *See also* Will to Live
    (WTL) study
    attachment and caregiving in, 48–49
    autonomy, challenges to, 68–69
    desire for death in, 78–79
    loss of personhood in care, 15
    mentalization in, 55–56
    mortality in, 14
    posttraumatic growth in, 88,
      89, 90, 91
    prognostic awareness, 71–72
    psychological interventions for,
      16, 99–102
    reclaiming identity, 61–62
    traumatic stress in patients
      with, 23–25
    treatment decisions, 68–72
caregivers
    attachment and caregiving, 48–49
    joint sessions with, 146, 164, 167–168
    Quality of Dying and Death
      study, 40–41
    traumatic stress symptoms in, 25–26
case examples
    beneath the surface, 193

changes in self and relationships,
    165–169
communication with healthcare
    providers, 159–164
considerate young woman, 190–192
facing the end, 193–194
finding a home, 185–188
focus on single domain in, 192
housecleaning and mortality, 188–190
professor, 183–185
recognizing tipping point, 194
self-knowledge, 192–193
single awareness, 195
spirituality or sense of meaning and
    purpose, 170–172
symptom management, 159–164
thinking of future, hope, and
    mortality, 173–175
CBTs (cognitive behavioral therapies),
    101–102
CEQ. *See* Clinical Evaluation
    Questionnaire
children, supporting, 168–169
Chochinov, H. M., 102
chronic living–dying phase, 32
Classen, C., 100
Clinical Evaluation Questionnaire (CEQ),
    221–222
    evaluating CALM therapy process
      with, 118, 179
    general discussion, 115–117
clinical trials, participation in, 69–70
clinicians, benefits of CALM training for,
    124–126
cognition and growth, 93
cognitive adaptation theory, 88–89
cognitive behavioral therapies (CBTs),
    101–102
cognitive existential group therapy, 141
cognitive mastery, 80–81
Colarusso, C. A., 142
collaborative care models, 102
collaborative relationships with
    healthcare providers, developing,
    162–163
communication with family and
    friends, 39
communication with healthcare
    providers
    case examples, 159–164

Printed in the USA
CPSIA information can be obtained
at www.ICGtesting.com
CBHW020122141223
2639CB00003B/4

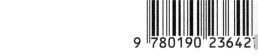